Praise for

exhausted

"We're facing an unprecedented healthcare crisis,
and much of it stems from the collapse of the energy
production systems of our cells. *Exhausted* is a timely
book that sheds light on the root of this epidemic. From
toxins to diet to exercise to sleep, Shojai and Polizzi do an
excellent job of bringing real solutions to the reader."

— Mark Hyman, M.D., *New York Times* best-selling author of *Food*;
Eat Fat, Get Thin; and *The Blood Sugar Solution*

"*Exhausted* presents the road map to refilling our drained
energy reserves and helping to prevent the degenerative
diseases that result from being in a state of sympathetic
depletion. It is a must-read for anyone who wants to
thrive in a sustainable way!"

— Tom O'Bryan, DC, CCN, DACBN, author of
The Autoimmune Fix

exhausted

exhausted

HOW TO REVITALIZE, RESTORE, AND RENEW YOUR ENERGY

NICK POLIZZI and PEDRAM SHOJAI, O.M.D.

HAY HOUSE, INC.
Carlsbad, California • New York City
London • Sydney • New Delhi

Copyright © 2020 by Rising Tide Productions, LLC

Published in the United States by: Hay House, Inc.: www.hayhouse.com®
Published in Australia by: Hay House Australia Pty. Ltd.: www.hayhouse.com.au
Published in the United Kingdom by: Hay House UK, Ltd.: www.hayhouse.co.uk
Published in India by: Hay House Publishers India: www.hayhouse.co.in

Indexer: J S Editorial, LLC
Cover design: Charles McStravick • *Interior design:* Nick C. Welch

Library of Congress Cataloging-in-Publication Data

Names: Polizzi, Nick, author. | Shojai, Pedram, author.
Title: Exhausted : how to revitalize, restore, and renew your energy / Nick Polizzi and Pedram Shojai.
Description: 1st edition. | Carlsbad : Hay House, Inc., 2020. | Includes bibliographical references.
Identifiers: LCCN 2020025767 | ISBN 9781401959005 (hardback) | ISBN 9781401959012 (ebook)
Classification: LCC HD69.T54 P645 2020 | DDC 650.1/1--dc23
LC record available at https://lccn.loc.gov/2020025767

Hardcover ISBN: 978-1-4019-5900-5
E-book ISBN: 978-1-4019-5901-2

10 9 8 7 6 5 4 3 2
1st edition, August 2020

Printed in the United States of America

To the seeker, who's been given answers but still feels exhausted, this is for you.

And to our wives, for being so patient, understanding, and supportive of us. We know how exhausting that can be.

contents

CHAPTER 1

Living in a Broken World

We have an epidemic in the modern world. Millions of us are waking up each and every morning feeling physically, mentally, emotionally, and spiritually drained. We simply don't have the energy we need to make it through our days.

Think of it this way. Imagine every morning when you open your eyes, you're given 100 units of energy to use. But before you even make it to the breakfast table, you burn 20 units off the top because of negative thought patterns, unresolved traumas, and stress in your environment (like a relationship that isn't working, or getting overstimulated by scary news headlines).

Now you're down to 80 units. That's a big problem because you need *100–120 units* to get through your commitments for the day. You may have kids who need parenting, errands to run, work to do, bosses and co-workers to appease, a spouse or partner who needs connection, aging parents who need checking in on . . . the list goes on.

So what do you do? You start borrowing energy from tomorrow to get through today by guzzling pots of coffee, cranking on sugary foods, cheating sleep, skipping exercise, and never slowing down. Just to make ends meet. Just to try to keep up with all the energy demands for the day.

But every morning you wake up with one or two fewer bars of energy. Now rinse and repeat every day, year after year. You keep waking up with one or two fewer bars of energy, but your commitments remain at 100–120.

You sink deeper into a pit of exhaustion. The anxiety that comes from having more to do than time to do it quickly becomes a heavy blanket of stress, weighing on you all the time. And as the stress overwhelms you, you become more sluggish.

We call this downward spiral *Deficit Spending*. Life has to be lived in balance, but you keep spending and depleting your energy without ever restoring it.

And you wind up exhausted.

The challenge with Deficit Spending is that the bill always comes due at some point. You may not feel the exhaustion in your twenties. Maybe you feel a little tired, but it's nothing an extra cup of coffee can't fix.

But flash forward 10 or 20 years, and eventually, your adrenals collapse. Your nervous system misfires. You can't get an erection. You can't get pregnant. You break out in acne. You gain weight. Your gut lining gets destroyed. You're bloated, gassy, or have weird bowel movements. You can't walk more than 10 minutes without wanting to keel over.

You live like this for a few years, and it doesn't take long before your immune system tanks, making you more susceptible to an opportunistic disease.

Exhaustion is often the gateway to bigger medical issues. Now your doctor runs some labs and pulls you aside, and regrets to inform you that you have diabetes, heart disease, multiple sclerosis, cancer, rheumatoid arthritis, Crohn's disease, or something else terrifying and debilitating. Cue the drugs. Now you can't live without the expensive pharmaceuticals and the miserable side effects they cause.

This is life in the modern world.

It sucks.

The very currency of life itself is *energy*. Everything else is secondary to this core biological need. You could have all the money in the world, a life chock full of exciting opportunities, a beautiful family, and a priceless circle of friends, but if you don't have the raw life-force energy to power you through this world, it all means nothing.

When you lack energy, you lack *life*.

When you hit this point, no wonder life feels so hard, heavy, dark, and overwhelming.

Now that we've shared the bad news, let's give you some good news. You don't have to live in a state of exhaustion. There is another way to experience your world, and we're going to show you how. In this book, we're going to give you some tools, techniques, strategies, and new mindsets to help you reverse your exhaustion, restore your energy, and get you feeling alive again.

We're going to help you boost your energy so you have the 100–120 units you need to power you through your day and commitments. We're going to stop the energy drains and replenish your reserves.

You can live a thriving life. In fact, you deserve it, so strap in as we take you on a ride through your exhaustion and to the other side—where joy, excitement, passion, purpose, and life await.

WHERE *EXHAUSTED* CAME FROM

Why should you let us be your guides on this trip? Well, we've dedicated our lives to helping people heal.

Pedram is a doctor of Oriental medicine, an ordained priest of the Yellow Dragon Monastery in China, an acclaimed qigong master, herbalist, documentary filmmaker, and founder of Well.org.

Nick produces feature-length documentaries about proven alternatives to conventional medicine, and is the founder of The Sacred Science, an organization dedicated to the research of ancient healing traditions.

We've both spent over two decades working in these fields, and exhaustion is one of the major themes that keeps popping up. Pedram ran into it often at his health clinic in Los Angeles. He treated patients who suffered from migraines and GI issues and so much more. Without fail, every single patient had one common symptom: exhaustion.

Many of their issues stemmed from being so exhausted that they didn't have enough energy for their bodies to biologically function right. After looking for the causes of their exhaustion and treating those, their other health issues cleared up.

While Pedram was busy treating patients, Nick was trekking through some of the world's most remote locations like the Amazon rainforest, the high Andes Mountains, and across the Sahara Desert. He was meeting, filming, and learning from indigenous shamans, medicine men, midwives, and other healers.

He has always been on the lookout for our cultural red flags and blind spots. For years, he was curious as to why we had such addictions to uppers and stimulants like coffee and energy drinks, and downers like alcohol and prescription drugs. He was always hunting for connections, and what did he find at the core? Glaring energy issues.

Every day we watch people of all ages, in all sorts of jobs and positions, married and single, with kids, grandkids, or without, utterly exhausted. They are dragging through life, and that pisses us off. People deserve better. They deserve to feel alive and thriving.

But there is a yawning gap in the health and wellness field when it comes to understanding and treating exhaustion. Modern medicine, especially Western trained doctors, really don't know how to address the issue. There's no magic pill that can treat it.

Fixing exhaustion often requires a multifaceted approach. It's about tweaking lifestyles, behaviors, and addressing underlying health issues unique to each person. It can take time, trial and error, patience, and what can feel like tough changes to diet, sleep, exercise, and stress management.

What happens to most of us? We end up wandering the exhaustion desert alone, living our lives assuming this level of fatigue—whether that's mental, emotional, physical, spiritual, all of it, or some combination—is just natural. We tell ourselves, it's part of our always-be-hustling, overworked, and success-driven culture. We assume it's simply a part of getting older. It happens to everyone, so what's the big deal?

But it is a huge deal. Not having the energy to power through your day means you don't show up as the husband or wife, the mother or father, the son or daughter, sister or brother, the best friend, the volunteer, the co-worker or boss that you want to be. It means you don't get to enjoy life, to feel the pleasure and exhilaration that comes from *being and feeling* alive.

When you restore your energy and you have enough units to meet all your commitments, you feel stronger, more focused, happier, more peaceful, and more filled with life.

Who doesn't want that?

LIVING IN A BROKEN WORLD

We're going to bust a lot of myths, misperceptions, unconscious thought patterns, and unintentional behaviors. We're also going to call bullshit on a lot of cultural and societal stories you've been force-fed.

We're calling BS right now on one of the biggest lies you've been told. It's the idea that you always have to do more. Run harder. Don't stop. Keep going. And when (not if) you become exhausted, "Congratulations! You are now part of the community," or "Oh, you feel tired? Well, too bad. Suck it up, because that's life. Everyone's exhausted."

No, everyone is not exhausted. No, stumbling through your day like a dead-eyed zombie is not living. It is not how life—how *your* life—is supposed to be.

You are living in a broken world with a flawed operating system.

In our Western culture, a lot of our self-worth is tied to *doing*. We tell ourselves that good parents stay involved. Good citizens volunteer. Good parishioners do bake sales. Good spouses have sex. Good employees respond to emails at 11 P.M. and on weekends. Good sons and daughters take their aging mothers and fathers to their doctors' appointments. Need we go on?

And this is on top of making sure we're wearing the "right" clothes, living in the "right" homes, driving the "right" vehicles, and acquiring all the other status symbols of life in the Western world. We end up living under these absurd expectations, running around, stressed out, disconnected from our bodies, minds, spirits, and each other.

You're exhausted, because you're living under unreasonable, unattainable, and impossible demands on your time and energy.

Our culture is dis-eased, and we're the only ones who don't know it. Both of us have spent a lot of time in other countries throughout the world and with many indigenous people who relish getting sunlight and stepping outside. The people we've met, observed, and learned from rest when they're tired and sleep more than four hours at night. They care about Mother Nature. They enjoy fantastic meals, cooked from whole foods, and eaten surrounded by their friends and family. They slow down. They move their bodies. They reconnect to their spirits or souls (or whatever term you want to use), and to each other.

They care about being an actual human being, not a human doing.

Let's pause for a second. Just sit with this idea for a moment. Being, *not* doing.

That's what we want to help you achieve in this book.

We know it's possible because we've both done it. We're not just two hippie-dippies living in the Rocky Mountains, in Colorado and Utah. We're busy dudes. We run multiple businesses, make documentary films, write books and blogs, and host podcasts, while also being husbands to our wives and dads to our young kiddos. We've got parents and siblings and friends we spend time with too. We go to the gym, go hiking, shoot hoops, practice kung fu and qigong, and fill our days with work, purpose, passion, family—with *life*.

We get shit done, but this is only possible because we've learned how to balance our energy economics. We use *and* replenish our energy stores. Both of us have built the right energy foundations to manage our days, time, and responsibilities. When you do that, then you have the fuel to live your life and truly enjoy yourself.

We've been exactly where you're sitting right now. We both had to learn the hard way that we weren't superheroes. At different times in our lives, we've found ourselves flat on our backs with no energy but tons of demands. We, too, have had to claw our way out of our own Deficit Spending. We did it, and so can you.

We know what's on the other side of your exhaustion—the promised land is real. We know what it takes—the time, patience, discipline, curiosity, commitment—to reverse exhaustion. And we know that when you do restore your energy, it is life altering.

YOUR EXHAUSTED ROAD TRIP

This book is not about our personal journeys—though we do share some of our stories and highlights.

This book is so much bigger than us. When we realized we wanted to write a book together on this topic, we knew it had to help people better understand what the hell was happening to their bodies, their minds, and their souls. We also wanted to give people different remedies grounded in science and backed by the world's leading experts to help them reset their energy economics.

We set out on a road trip—camera and film crews in hand—and interviewed more than 60 of the world's leading health, wellness and fitness experts, doctors, functional medicine practitioners, and top researchers. We spoke with incredible people such as Dr. Mark Hyman, Ari Whitten, Dr. David Perlmutter, Dr. Kellyann Petrucci, Dr. Datis Kharrazian, Dr. Leigh Erin Connealy, Dr. Joe Mercola, Magdalena Wszelaki, Dr. Darin Ingels, Dr. Robert Rountree, Ben Greenfield, and so many more.

Exhausted is their collected wisdom.

What you're about to read comes from their research and work helping thousands of patients heal their exhaustion and regain their energy and life force. It includes their best tips, techniques, and insights on the story of exhaustion. *Exhausted* is also everything we've learned on our own journeys to and through exhaustion, and the work we've both done in the health and wellness space for over two decades.

We're taking you on a road trip that spans the next eight chapters. Each chapter is both a major cause of exhaustion and a path back from the brink. The topics include: diet and nutrition, the gut and immune system, exercise and movement, sleep and recovery, toxins, adrenals and hormones, the brain, and spiritual health.

These eight topics will form the foundation for your energy. When you master these areas, you master your energy.

We've divided each chapter into four core parts. We open with a case study to illustrate the problem you're facing before moving into some possible energy drains that could be contributing to your exhaustion. Next, we offer some key tests that you can do on your own, or that a doctor may order to help assess the problem. From there, we explore some promising remedies with you, before closing each chapter with a one-week personal challenge designed to help you move your energy in the right direction.

A big part of this book is about bringing more awareness and understanding to potential causes and solutions to help restore your energy. Often, there's a lot of mystery around exhaustion. Most people—doctors too—have no idea where it comes from or even why someone's energy is gone.

As you'll find out, exhaustion has many root causes. You could have gut issues, hidden infections, exposure to toxins, or adrenal and hormone challenges from eating the wrong foods or poor sleep.

There are very real physiological reasons why you're exhausted, and our intention is to let you see behind the curtain of your exhaustion and to increase your awareness about what's going on inside your body.

Functional Medicine Understood

This book is meant to guide you on your exhaustion journey. For some people, they may need more help. Finding the right medical ally is very important. A general practitioner may or may not be the right stop.

Most Western trained M.D.s are taught to pinpoint a disease and prescribe the right medication, drug, or procedure. But exhaustion doesn't present like, say, cancer or diabetes. There is no drug or pill that can reverse this.

Instead, you may want to consider seeking out an integrative and/or functional medicine professional. Functional medicine has grown in the last decade, because it supports the whole person, and seeks to find the root of illnesses, especially chronic ones. Functional care and treatment plans are typically customized to fit the unique needs of the patient.

Many tests that we cover in this book can be ordered through a functional medicine practitioner. In fact, many of these tests won't ever be offered by a general practitioner.

Just as the reasons why you're exhausted are varied, so too are the remedies. Throughout this book, we're going to identify the best practices that are scientifically proven to help you feel better and have more energy. Upon first glance, some of these might feel like a step backward. Trust it.

To have more energy, there are some things you'll need to correct and adjust. As you do so, you'll start having more enthusiasm and clarity in your life. You'll start managing your time better, and you'll likely find that you get things done right the first time.

Right now, your exhaustion might have you reading over lines, forgetting your keys, and going back to the grocery store three times each week. When you have more energy and clarity, you have your game together better and are actually *better at life*. That's the consistent feedback we get from people who snap out of the trance and decide to heal their exhaustion. Fix your energy economics and stop being broke!

We know, you probably want a 30-day or a 21-step action plan to reverse your exhaustion. Hell, we'd love to see one of those too. "Just do X, Y, and Z and you'll be recovered in no time!" is a pretty standard line in the health and wellness industry. By all means, that might work on certain health issues. But not with exhaustion.

Your body is unique, and your path to healing and restoring your energy is too. We can, and will, lead you to different pathways that will restore your life force, but ultimately you have to discover what remedies, in what combination, and in what order will work for you. There's a big experiential component to this book. Trial and error are real when it comes to fixing your energy.

We're not trying to scare or discourage you. Quite the opposite. We want to inspire you to control your destiny. We want you to reconnect and learn to listen to your body, and understand what it needs and when. As Dr. David Perlmutter, a board-certified neurologist and fellow of the American College of Nutrition, told us, "Simple steps can go a long way to creating a pattern that feeds forward, allowing you to leverage more and more of these ideas to create a much better, more energetic life."[1]

We've written this book so each chapter builds on the next. But if you want to skip around, reading this more like a choose your own adventure, have at it. This is your journey. Own it.

As you read, stay curious about discovering the causes of your exhaustion. Stay determined to heal and restore your life force. And stay proud for taking this step toward reversing your exhaustion. It takes work, patience, strength, and courage, but the rewards are so worth it.

We know you can do this.

Now, let's go kick your exhaustion in the ass.

CHAPTER 2

Diet and Nutrition

Katie took her health very seriously. It mattered—after all, she was a personal stylist and prided herself on looking good.

She had seen a registered dietician and had tried several different nutrition strategies in an attempt to live healthy. She ate a low-fat diet and tracked her calories religiously, keeping them to about 1,800 per day, because at 30 years old, she wanted to lose weight and fit into her size-6 jeans again. Every morning, noon, and night, she diligently weighed, measured, and portioned every ounce that went into her body, according to the guidelines she'd been given.

Katie was doing all the right things.

But her energy levels kept plummeting while the scale kept rising. She had always yo-yo'd a bit through her twenties, but in the last couple of years, she had watched her weight go up by 10 pounds, then 15, then 20, then 25. Nothing she was doing was working and she was exhausted.

Soon, Katie started to lose her confidence. She had always loved helping her clients make empowering choices and look and feel their best. But if *she* wasn't looking good or feeling good, how could she claim she could help someone else? She was embarrassed, and afraid, because she had no idea what to do.

THE PROBLEM

We're starting our exhaustion journey with diet and nutrition, because that's the foundation for your vitality.

Energy cannot be made. It has to be converted from one form into another. Enter food. Our bodies take what we eat and convert it into energy that our cells then use to fire our brains, power our hearts, move our legs and arms, and do the millions of other small and large tasks needed for us to live.

Take the word *calorie*. It's a scientific term for a unit of energy. It means the amount of heat needed to raise the temperature of one gram of water by one degree Celsius. In layman's terms, it means the amount of energy you get from what you consume.

Food is our fuel in life, but let's be honest. How often during your day do you pause to ask, "Hey, what should I eat to power my body?" Probably rarely to never. That's because we aren't taught to think about food as fuel or to see it as the life-giving sustenance that it is.

For many of us, food is something we live in fear of. We're afraid of eating too much or eating the wrong foods. We're so busy chasing the latest diet craze, and trying to keep our bodies looking attractive or dropping the number on our scales, that we're trapped in dysfunctional relationships with food, and by extension with ourselves.

Food has become such a loaded, toxic part of our lives that it no longer energizes us. It only drags us further into the dark recesses of exhaustion.

It's time to fix this and return to what food is all about—fueling your body, mind, and heart so you have the energy you need to live a big life.

Food has such a huge impact on your energy that we're devoting two chapters to it. In Chapter 3, we'll look at how food intolerances, allergies, and digestion and immune system issues may be hijacking your energy, and what you can do to heal those problems.

But in this chapter, we're starting with the basics. We're diving into some of the universal truths about food. We're also tackling some of the fundamental principles of diet and nutrition. Our goal is to cut through the noise and distraction to help you build a food foundation that's *right for you*.

We're going to look at how your body transforms food into energy, the fuel sources it uses like proteins, fats, and carbohydrates, how following the "right" diets might be sabotaging your energy levels, what minerals and nutrients you need, and how you may have lost your connection to the true meaning of food and eating.

As you make your way through, be curious and open to looking at your diet and nutrition in a different light. Be willing to let go of any preconceived ideas you have around food like what you should eat, how much, and when. Food is not your enemy. It is one of your biggest allies on your quest to regaining and maintaining your vitality.

Food is how you get the energy you need to live. So don't fear it. It's to be celebrated and enjoyed. It truly is the bounty of the gods. It is life giving and life sustaining.

THE ENERGY DRAINS

Energy Drain #1: You're Fueling with Too Many Carbs

In its most basic terms, food is trapped sunlight stuck in chemical bonds.

We know that probably sounds confusing, so let's go back to the beginning of time for a quick history lesson. Miraculously, life on the third rock from the sun began with the fungus kingdom. Next the plant kingdom showed up and it figured out how to photosynthesize, which means that plants learned how to take the light from the sun and combine it with water and gasses in the air to make glucose—a form of sugar. The plants then used that sugar to keep growing. They actually fed themselves.

Eventually, mammals came along, and they started eating the plants, which contained all that trapped sunlight and energy. Next other mammals adapted to eat other animals, which had feasted on the plants. Then we, *Homo sapiens*, arrived and started eating plants and animals.

We get our energy by unlocking that trapped sunlight through a two-step process: *digestion and metabolism.*

Step 1: Digestion. The digestion process breaks down our food into what's called micronutrients and macronutrients. *Micronutrients* are the vitamins and minerals like magnesium, iron, B_{12} vitamins, and so many more that our bodies need in smaller doses to stay healthy and function optimally. *Macronutrients* are the carbohydrates, proteins, and fats that our bodies need in much larger quantities.

Step 2: Metabolism. We use macronutrients to generate the fuel that powers our cells. So once the food we've eaten has been broken down, then it heads to our small intestines (also known as the gut lining). From there, the macronutrients pass through the gut lining to enter the blood stream. Once in the blood stream, the macronutrients get carried to the trillions of cells in our bodies.

Waiting in our cells for the macronutrients are the *mitochondria.* Mitochondria are the powerhouses. They are the energy producers. They take the macronutrients, and through a complex process that involves oxygen, chemical reactions, and lots of micronutrients, they transform the food we eat into *ATP (adenosine triphosphate).*

ATP holds the energy that powers all the trillions of cells in your body.

Mitochondria play a starring role in the story of exhaustion, and are key to correcting your energy economics. As evolutionist Lynn Margulis explained in her widely accepted theory, our mitochondria used to live outside our bodies billions of years ago. It was then that our granddaddy cells struck a gangbuster deal with the mitochondria. The mitochondria would live inside our cells in a symbiotic relationship. In exchange for room and board, the mitochondria agreed to make energy for our cells.

This was life's true gold rush. Before the mitochondria moved inside, our cells were only cranking out about two ATP units from our food. But with our cells' new BFFs, that energy production accelerated to about *18 ATP units.*

This enabled us to quickly grow bigger, faster, stronger, and smarter until we became the complex beings populating the earth today.

To make ATP, your mitochondria can use any of the macronutrients you ingest—proteins, fats, or carbohydrates. But not all the macronutrients were created equal. You actually get more bang for your buck when your body runs off fat than from protein. There's simply more energy stored in fat. Fat has about nine calories per gram compared to carbohydrates and protein, which have about four calories per gram.[1]

Unfortunately, most of us in the Western world don't fuel our bodies with fat or protein. Instead, we use *fast carbohydrates*—the worst fuel source. "Carbs" are a broad category. They include everything from "slow carbs" found in things like organic fruits and veggies, wild grains, beans, and seeds to the not-so-great "fast carbs" found in enriched white flour, white pasta, and sweeteners like high-fructose corn syrup.

Fast carbs come from the foods we love to eat, but know we shouldn't, at least in the quantities we usually consume them. They include the oh-so-tempting, and oh-so-addictive fast foods, fried foods, muffins, donuts, pastries, white bread, ice cream, pretzels, peanut-butter cookies, croissants, chips, candy . . . do we really need to keep going?

No one expects you to be a Puritan and never indulge. But most of us—and we're both raising our hands here—have at some point overindulged beyond what our bodies can handle. When we fuel ourselves primarily with fast carbs, we end up losing more energy than we create.

When carbohydrates (fast and slow) are digested, they break down into glucose, a type of sugar. That glucose then floods the bloodstream, raising blood sugar levels. This causes a spike in the hormone insulin. Insulin acts as a messenger, showing up to knock on the front door of your cells saying, "Hey, open up. We've got a sugar delivery for the mitochondria." The cells open the front door, and into the cells goes all that sugar.

Fast carbs are so named because our cells will quickly burn through the energy created from this fuel source. Then they need more. It's throwing kindling on a fire. You digest and burn through fast carbs so quickly that you need a constant supply to keep your fire stoked.

This is the sugar rush/sugar crash. Once all that sugar is gone, we're left feeling tired and lethargic until we get our next hit. We've all experienced this. Think about a typical day. At about 7 A.M., you grab coffee, maybe a double caramel macchiato, and a muffin that you eat on the way to work. Your energy spikes, but by 10 A.M. you're feeling a little groggy, maybe irritable. Maybe you start sweating as your heart rate rises.

Uh-oh. Your sugar is dropping, and your brain knows it, and it's not okay. Like the sugar addict your brain has become, it needs its next fix. Yes, we called it an "addict." That's exactly what it is. Sugar actually triggers the same center in your brain as cocaine.[2] Yes, *that* cocaine. To soothe the shakes and sweats, you need another hit, so you reach for another quick energy pick-me-up. Up your blood sugar climbs. You're feeling more alert and happier. For a few hours, you're in the clear.

Lunch time rolls around, and man, are you starving. You're feeling a little angry too. Your belly's talking to you, and your energy is getting low. The crashing is coming fast, so you grab a whole-grain sandwich, bag of chips, maybe a "healthy" soda, and bam! Like magic, up your sugar and energy go again.

By 3 P.M., you're in serious trouble. You're slumping over your desk, exhausted, barely able to keep your eyes open. Your sugar level has crashed. Thank God you have that secret stash of M&M's in your drawer, or maybe that gluten-free bar that's laced with sugar. If you've already gone over to the dark side, that's when the energy drink comes out.

You pop the snack and get a little energy burst that holds you until dinner, which is pasta and turkey meatballs, a tossed salad with ranch dressing, and a glass of pinot noir. If you're still awake by 10 P.M. (which, of course you are), then you're crashing, and that tub of chocolate ice cream in the freezer is hard to resist, or perhaps the gluten-free, dairy-free tub of "healthy" sugar that still fucks you up all the same.

All day long, you've ridden this roller coaster where your blood sugar and energy levels rocket up, then crash, rocket up and crash, rocket up and crash. This ride alone is a huge drain on your energy, not to mention the pressure you're placing on your organs to keep digesting.

When you're fueling with the fast carbs and eating all the time, you can also hit a point where your cells actually don't need more energy. But you still have all that sugar from the carbs in your system. Now any extra calories you consume fly past the mitochondria and head straight for your fat cells for a little rainy-day storage. We're talking about the fat you see on your waist, butt, thighs, and all of those places you hate to look at.

And when you fuel with fast carbs year after year, then you're not just battling exhaustion, you also place yourself at serious risk for more health complications. You could develop type 2 diabetes, cardiovascular issues, and high blood pressure.

Energy Drain #2: You're Missing Key Nutrients

Your body needs a lot of micronutrients to function. That's key nutrients and minerals that you need in smaller doses compared to macronutrients. Micronutrients do a lot for your body. They help digest macronutrients, ensure your organs function properly, and keep you feeling energized and healthy.

When you're missing key vitamins and minerals, it can wreck your energy levels. In the Remedies section, we'll share some tips on how to get these levels up if you're deficient. But for now, let's take a look at some of the MVPs in the vitamin and mineral world.

Magnesium. Magnesium is the one thing that binds to ATP and allows it to do its job. Without adequate magnesium, the over 300 reactions in the human body that need ATP don't work, and you'll feel exhausted. You don't need a blood test to know when you're low in magnesium. If you experience fatigue, eye-twitching, cramping, racing thoughts that don't stop, headaches, insomnia, or restless legs, get yourself some magnesium.

Iron. Mitochondria also require oxygen to make ATP. Iron is part of the heme that becomes hemoglobin, which is responsible for carrying oxygen from the lungs to each and every cell of the body. Once both oxygen and iron are in the cell, they are used in the actual process of making ATP from your food energy.

No energy can be made without oxygen. And there is no oxygen in your cells without iron.

Is it any wonder that the primary symptom of iron deficiency, which is anemia, is fatigue? Imagine trying to hold your breath for more than a minute. How do you feel? You have a hard time functioning without oxygen, don't you? Well, so do your cells.

Your doctor can test you for anemia, so if you don't know your iron status, and you've suffered from fatigue for longer than you wish, you may have an easy fix to a complex problem. It's worth getting checked out.

B vitamins (specifically B_{12}). B_{12} is needed for forming the red blood cells that carry hemoglobin and oxygen around the body. When you are insufficient in B_{12}, your red blood cells are larger, misshaped, and not very good at carrying oxygen in hemoglobin.

Anybody can wind up with a B_{12} deficiency, but vegans and vegetarians are particularly at risk. Meat, poultry, fish, scallops, yogurt, milk, and eggs are good sources of B_{12}. While a plant-based diet has some terrific benefits, if you're on one, you need to monitor your B_{12} carefully, since there is no bioavailable B_{12} in plants. You may need to incorporate supplements.

Energy Drain #3:
You're Trying to Keep Up with the "Right" Diet

Which diet is the "right" diet? How are you supposed to choose between Paleo or Keto? Do you count calories? Should you stop eating meat and become a vegetarian? Should you just send in a check to become a lifetime member of the vegan club? How about going gluten-free? Hell, maybe you should just hunt elk with your bare hands and beat your chest.

What if there was no such thing as the perfect, universal diet for reversing exhaustion and gaining energy? What if the perfect diet is like finding the perfect partner?

The diet isn't perfect, but it's perfect for you.

That's the idea shared by numerous experts like Ari Whitten, an energy and fatigue expert, who told us there isn't a standard diet they prescribe to their exhausted patients. "Within the realm of nutrition, there's a lot of debate, dietary dogmas, and camps of people saying, 'Oh, everybody needs to go vegan. Everybody needs to go low carb. Everybody needs to go low fat. Everybody needs to go paleo or keto.' In terms of the science, there isn't a specific diet that's best for fatigue," he explained. "There isn't even a specific correlation between any optimal macronutrient ratio as being the critical or best for people with fatigue."[3]

When we heard this, we both felt relieved. Like we were given permission to not jump on the paleo or keto bandwagon unless we wanted—no disrespect to our paleo and keto brothers and sisters. These are just two of the most popular diets talked about in the health world today.

It's hard to walk away from what's "hot" or the latest 90-day diet craze promoted by some tabloid and guaranteed to help restore your energy and help you lose 20 pounds too. We get the temptation to jump onboard the diet-craze train. We want solutions. We want to feel better. We want plans that spell out to a T what to eat, when to eat, and how much to eat.

Here's the thing: diets come and go. Ten years ago, the Atkins Diet and the South Beach Diet were all the rage. Even foods once deemed off limits are coming back in good graces (hello, egg yolks).

Diets are personal. You have to experiment to find what restores your energy, and what robs you. We know people who swear by going vegan. We know others who have cut out all dairy and are living their best lives. We know others who have no restrictions and just eat in moderation. We know some people who once swore by eating vegetarian, who have now added some lean meat into their diets.

Diets are so varied when it comes to what works for some people and what doesn't for others that for us to stand here and tell you that without a doubt you should "eat this and only this" would be absurd. Plus, what works for you today may not work tomorrow. Your diet has a lot to do with how much exercise and movement you get (see Chapter 4 for more on this topic) too. Hell, even your sleep plays a role in how you're digesting and metabolizing your food (check out Chapter 5 for more info on sleep).

Your diet and nutrition are constant evolution at its finest. But if you're constantly jumping on the latest diet craze, then you risk draining your energy instead of revitalizing it. You risk never really tapping into what *you* need to eat and when.

Yet jumping from one diet to the next, trying desperately to keep up with the *wisdom du jour,* is where so many of us live. Our intentions are honorable. We want to feel better, to feel more energized, and probably to lose weight too. But diet hopping is a path to exhaustion.

Energy Drain #4: You're Not Eating Enough *Slow* Carbs

Earlier in this chapter we fileted carbohydrates, making them sound like the devil's creation. Now we'll play his advocate: *you still need to eat your carbs.*

Not all carbs are created equal, and yet all the fad diets these days are pointing to a low-carb/high-fat diet, often with a lot of fasting mixed throughout. Contrary to popular belief, the low-carb diet isn't new—it's been used to treat epilepsy in children for over 100 years—and it does this *well.* But that doesn't mean it's for everyone.

While many of the core tenets of new diets like keto and paleo are good, many folks find them very hard to follow because they require extremely disciplined eating—with a big emphasis on red meats and fatty foods to make up for the absence of carbohydrates. (By the way—carbs normally comprise 50 percent of the calories we eat, so subbing them out with bacon and ghee is a heavy lift.)

After adopting one of the new fad diets mentioned above, many people stop eating even the bare minimum amount of carbs. And they get lost in the all-or-nothing space of thinking all grains, breads, and pastas are bad, when, in fact, sometimes we need the carbs from these foods—whole grains are especially good—for an energy boost.

When you're not eating enough carbs, that can affect your sleep, gut health, and energy levels.

Energy Drain #5: Your Gratitude Is Gone

You are a part of the natural world. You are connected to all life forms on this planet, and as such, your body is subject to the same rules, and freedoms, that are true for all life.

All life needs to eat. All life needs to process what it's consumed to make the energy needed to heal, to reproduce, to keep growing, to survive, *to live*. You are not a plant, capable of absorbing sunlight, mixing it with water and carbon dioxide and making your own food.

To power your body, you must unlock those sun packets stored in other living creatures. To live, you must consume the life force and energy from others. Does that make you uncomfortable? Good. You should be.

Food isn't just some abstract idea. It's not a bunch of calories that you manage. It isn't just a thing you walk into the grocery store, buy, and come home and cook. When you eat, you are consuming another life, another creature's life force, because for some reason, your life was deemed more important.

Food is the sacrifice you bring to the altar of life. Another life form, be it a cabbage, an apple, a cow, a pig, a fish, laid down its life so you could continue to live.

Our ancestors had so many rituals connected to hunting and taking of another life's being. Many indigenous tribes throughout the world still do. But we have largely forgotten this sacred contract we have with Mother Earth, God, or whatever divine being you want to call it.

When we foraged or hunted for food and brought some home, we celebrated. We gave thanks to the animal or plant for laying down its life so we, and our families, could go on living. That gratitude alone upped our energy, reinforcing this unseen power inside of us.

But now we're terrified of food. We're afraid it will make us fat, or gassy, or bloated. We often take for granted that it will always just be there, and we forget—intentionally or unintentionally—that it, too, once moved through the world, living, breathing, eating, being a part of nature.

When we forget these connections, we lose our energy a little more every day.

Personal Quest (Nick)

When I was in my late thirties, I decided to get into better shape. Really, I was just trying to figure out how not to get old so fast. (Midlife crisis? Maybe.) So I went on a gluten-free diet. I ate tons of meat, greens, and some potatoes now and then.

I got ripped, and I felt great.

The diet was easy to stick with too. No gluten became my way of life.

But there's an incubation period for physical changes, and it can take some time for any issues to make themselves known to us. Over the next two to three years, I realized that I was having serious energy issues. I didn't get it. I was eating well, sleeping, exercising, and meditating, and I wasn't drinking coffee. Why was I feeling like shit?

One morning, I woke up and my family and I were supposed to go hiking, but I was so exhausted. I thought, *I want to be a great dad today. I don't want to let them down,* but I wasn't sure I had it in me.

Instead of brushing aside my exhaustion or saying "sorry, kids," I tuned in to my body. I asked myself, *What do you need right now?* To my surprise, my body demanded a goddamn sandwich. My boys eat this amazing Portuguese bread, so I slathered two thick slices with mayonnaise and cheese, threw on some salami, and just said, "The hell with it."

About halfway through the sandwich, my energy shot up. It was like I'd had a cup of coffee. It made zero sense, and it went against just about every diet there is right now. But I went on my hike, feeling awesome, and we all had a great day.

A week later I talked with my buddy Chris Kresser, a functional medicine practitioner, and told him about the sandwich. He laughed and said that about half of his patients who suffer from exhaustion also experience what he called *unintentional carb decrease.*

We have so many diets flying at us, and many limit carbs. But 50 percent of the calories we consume should be carbs. Gluten-free does not mean carb-free. Some people need the occasional slice of bread—whether it's gluten-free or not.

TESTS

A doctor is likely to test your nutrient levels. They'll want to know if your body is absorbing what it needs. Here are a few tests that your doctor may recommend.

Nutrition Panel

You can be deficient in vitamins, amino acids, fatty acids, and minerals. Instead of randomly picking a supplement, this can help you target what your body needs to feel energized. You'll want to get panels like ION or NutrEval, as they cover all the bases.

Normal Nutrient Test

Zinc, magnesium, and iron are all crucial to your energy, and can all be measured by a normal CBC (complete blood count) test and simple add-ons. For iron, your functional medicine practitioner may do a blood test to look at your red blood cells (RBC), mean corpuscular hemoglobin concentration (MCHC), hematocrit, total iron, ferritin, iron saturation, and total iron binding capacity (TIBC).

Your doctor can look at B_{12} levels by drawing your blood and looking at your MCV (mean corpuscular volume), and your MCHC (mean corpuscular hemoglobin concentration). If your MCV is elevated and your MCHC is normal, you may have an issue with B_{12} deficiency.

Another way to examine B_{12} is to run a test called *methylmalonic acid*, or *MMA*. This marker appears to be more accurate in determining B_{12} deficiencies than the serum B_{12} that is often run in doctors' offices.

Acetylcarnitine is another important nutrient that your doctor will look for by running nutrient panels like the ION and NutrEval tests. They'll likely look for specific markers called *adipate* and *suberate*. If one or both of these are elevated, you may have a deficiency of this important nutrient carrier.

THE ENERGY REMEDIES

Energy Remedy #1: Change Your Fuel Source

The cliché "you are what you eat" holds so much truth. More importantly, your body runs on the fuel you give it, so the first step toward reversing your exhaustion is to ask, "What fuel do I primarily use?"

Do you supply your body with fresh, whole, organic vegetables and fruits, and grains and fibers? Are you eating lean and clean, humanely raised, grass-fed, and organic meat? Are you running off fast or slow carbs?

It's time to dig into your diet and bring more awareness to what you're fueling with. We know we're not breaking new ground here when we say, "Cut back on the fast carbs." For decades, the medical community has beat the drum that we need to reduce our fast carb and sugar intake.

Yet despite the information, many of us continue to eat too many fast carbs (sugar and saturated fat too) and not enough slow carbs. In a recent U.S. government study that spanned 16 years (from 1999–2016), researchers found that Americans got 42 percent of their daily energy intake from fast carbs.[4] The same study found that Americans got over 10 percent of their energy from saturated fats—including fatty beef, pork, high-fat dairy, and fried foods.[5] When it came to eating more slow carbs, Americans increased their consumption by only one percent.[6]

Most of us know what we need to do; it's the *how* that mystifies us. Let's start by banishing any self-judgment or shame around what we've been eating. Think about your food as being your fuel (because it is). Next, let's focus on switching your fuel source. You don't have to do a complete 180 overnight. Make small adjustments to your diet and food choices.

You can gradually and continually ween your body off fast carbs and onto the slower ones with lean protein and healthy fat.

Here are a few tips to help you make a smooth, and steady, adjustment.

Track What You Eat

We want you to take a close, honest look at your diet and consider which macronutrients you are eating the most. We're both big fans of tracking what you eat. You can do this on your phone with an app, or go old school and grab a notebook or open a document on your computer or tablet, and record what you eat, when you're eating, and how much you eat during the day. There are apps like bitesnap (getbitesnap.com) where all you have to do is take a picture, and the app counts the calories and breaks down the nutrients in the food.

Consider writing down how you feel after a meal too. Note if you feel gassy, bloated, or have stomach pains after a meal. Track if you feel energized (you should) or if you feel like you need a nap.

Do this for a week, so you get a real accounting for your diet, and it will help you find the right macronutrient balance. It will also help you with what we're covering in Chapter 3—food intolerances and allergies. Many people have food intolerances, and tracking their diets can help them decipher what foods they may need to omit or limit.

Don't Drink Your Energy

Are you drinking your energy, living off energy drinks and other beverages? If so, stop. Think about it this way. You can eat an orange, and it's great. Sure, it's got sugar, but it's also got a ton of vitamins and fiber. But if you drink a glass of orange juice, it's just highly concentrated sugar without the fiber. Your body will immediately work to convert the sugar to ATP, but it can't always keep up with the huge load in juices, so you are likely to convert some of that into fat. This is also going to cause a big blood sugar spike that sends you on a roller coaster. Eat the orange, skip the OJ.

And please, for the love of all that is holy, stay away from those Frappuccinos. A 12-ounce caramel Frappuccino has *38 grams of sugar with most of it coming from high-fructose corn syrup.* Don't do that to yourself.

If anything—anything at all—contains high-fructose corn syrup (HFCS), back away slowly. HFCS causes intestinal permeability and affects your liver, which will cause insulin resistance, which then leads to type 2 diabetes and all sorts of nasty side effects that can destroy your energy and body.

Stabilize Your Blood Sugar Levels

This isn't something that will happen overnight, but just getting off the fast carbs and adding the slow carbs, mixed with lean protein, and healthy fats can go a long way to increasing your energy and getting your body used to burning different fuel sources.

How do you transition from fast carbs that might be causing your blood sugar to spike? Try this four-step process:

Step 1: Every three hours, eat a mixture of the macronutrients—some protein, fat, and slow carbohydrates.

Step 2: The protein should be equivalent to the palm of your hand. This could mean a couple of eggs (yolks too) or four or five ounces of lean meat.

Step 3: You should eat a couple of tablespoons of fat. This could be coconut oil, butter, nuts, seeds, or half an avocado.

Step 4: Throw in some good slow carbs like a handful of fresh or frozen blueberries, or other vegetables or fruit.

Try this for about a week and track your energy. See how you feel throughout the day.

If you really want to have some fun with a personal experiment, you can grab a glucometer from your local grocery store and see exactly what your blood sugar is before and after eating certain foods. This can be a real eye opener and an inspiration to choose slow carbs and other healthy options.

Energy Remedy #2: Get Nutrient Rich

Your first step is to get those optimal nutrient panels, so you know what you're dealing with and what kinds of foods or supplements you may need to add to your diet. Ideally, you'd also work with a medical professional like a functional medicine doctor who could help guide you toward the right doses of a supplement for your body. That's a far better, and safer, approach than running to the health food store, buying a supplement off the shelf, and just popping pills.

We're identifying some of the top energy nutrients that many doctors will look at. At the very least, ensuring you have a balanced and varied diet that contains more nutrients is a safe road to take.

Here are some of the nutrients you want to make sure you have in your diet.

Magnesium

If you're low in magnesium, start with eating foods that are high in magnesium, like beans, greens, nuts, seeds, and meat—though, you'll want to make sure you have the stomach acid and enzymes to digest it. If your numbers aren't going up quickly enough, you can supplement.

There are a few options for magnesium supplements:

1. Magnesium Citrate helps keep the bowels regular.

2. Magnesium Glycinate is better for those with sensitive guts or who are prone to diarrhea (if this is you, don't take magnesium citrate, okay?).

3. Magnesium Threonate, which is helpful if you're experiencing some memory loss or concentration issues with your low magnesium.

Iron

Foods that are high in iron include spinach, legumes (which have to be soaked well), pumpkin seeds, red meat, quinoa, broccoli, dark chocolate, turkey, shellfish, liver and organ meats—though, again, make sure your body is digesting them properly before relying on them.

If you need to supplement, be careful how much you're taking. High doses of iron can be toxic, so seek guidance from a doctor. Ferrous iron is more easily absorbed by the body, but if you have stomach upset, you can try heme iron polypeptides.[7]

B_{12}

Many of the foods that are high in iron are also high in B_{12}—meats, especially organ meats, and many kinds of fish (though watch the mercury and other contaminants). Nutritional yeast is also a good alternative, but if you're vegan or vegetarian, you may need to take a supplement.

Acetylcarnitine

Fueling your body with healthy fats is a great source of energy. Fat contains nine calories per gram, while carbs and proteins contain four. But these calories from fat can only be utilized if they're correctly digested and transported to your mitochondria.

To get the fat to the mitochondria requires a special transport protein, called the *carnitine shuttle*. As its name implies, a key ingredient is carnitine. If your body is low in a specific form of carnitine, called *acetylcarnitine*, you may not be getting as much energy from fat as you could, and this will leave you tired.

Because acetylcarnitine and lysine (which the body uses to make carnitine) are most often found in meat, vegans and vegetarians may be at risk for deficiencies here. In order for your body to produce it in sufficient amounts, you actually need plenty of vitamin C[8] and other nutrients like B_{12}, iron, B_6, and niacin. If you really need dietary supplements, you may consider acetylcarnitine, but check with your doctor first about how much you need to take. You can also try to naturally boost your vitamin C with broccoli, brussels sprouts, cauliflower, green and red peppers, spinach, cabbage, other leafy greens, sweet and white potatoes, tomatoes, winter squash, oranges, strawberries, and pink grapefruit.

Coenzyme Q10

Coenzyme Q10 (CoQ10) is the *only* nutrient that sits in something called the *electron transport chain*. This is the last step in producing the majority of a cell's ATP. When CoQ10 is low, it can limit energy production.

CoQ10 is found in many of the foods already listed—organ meats, fatty fish, fruits, vegetables, legumes, and seeds. With the exception of animal hearts and livers, it is very difficult to bring CoQ10 levels up by diet alone. In many cases, supplements can work well.

Energy Remedy #3: Find Your Perfect Diet

You will always find someone who raves about the newest diet fad and all the benefits. There's truth to these stories, but it's up to you to determine what foods work for your body. Sometimes that means trial and error. If you want to try a fad diet, go for it. But be aware while you're doing it.

As we mentioned with your fuel sources, if you go on a specific diet, it's wise to keep track of how you feel, your energy levels, and other effects. Act like a scientist and record your observations. This isn't a useless practice. It's a great way to dial in to what you're eating and how that food makes you feel. There really is no one diet that works for everyone, so you have to find what's right for you.

We know you're bombarded with different diets, so we're giving you a quick primer on some of the popular crazes we're seeing today. We'll let you be the judge on what to try, if any. Just remember, it's always okay to pass. Just because your pal Sam has gone Paleo doesn't mean you have to. There is absolutely no shame in walking away from the masses and listening to your own inner voice that tells you what foods to eat and what diet fits you best.

This takes courage, for sure, but you'll be one step closer to fixing your exhaustion.

Paleo

Paleo diet makes a lot of sense to us. Eat foods like we used to eat back in the days of hunting and gathering? Foods that our immune system recognizes? Foods that our digestive system was built on? Hell yes!

The trouble with Paleo is not actually the diet. It's with the folks who focus only on the *hunting* part of hunting and gathering. Yes, our ancestors hunted elk with their bare hands and a spear. But you know what else they did? They foraged. They ate vegetables and nuts and fruits and fiber. Cavemen didn't eat just meat, because meat was actually really dangerous to try to get.

You know what else they didn't eat? Butter. No other animal on this planet consumes another animal's breast milk, much less distills the fat from it and smears that fat all over everything. (Just saying.)

If you're going to eat Paleo, *actually* eat Paleo. Consume meat, but do it sparingly, treating it as something valuable, something that took a lot of effort to get. And make sure your diet includes fruits, vegetables, and nuts in great quantities—those were a lot easier to come by for your hunter-gatherer ancestors.

Finally, don't just eat Paleo, *live* Paleo. This doesn't mean you need to go hunt that elk, but you should go for a jog, running like you had to try to catch an animal faster than you, and lift weights like you had to haul buckets of water from the river. And drink lots of that water too.

Keto

Ketosis is when our bodies switch from burning carbohydrates and sugars as fuel to using fat. The keto diet is geared toward encouraging your body to stick with this process. It has become hugely popular in the last few years. This is a high-fat, moderate protein, low-carb, no sugar diet.

For certain people, ketogenic diets can be fantastic. Studies are showing keto is good for reversing diabetes and getting people off insulin.[9] When you don't have high blood sugar spikes, your pancreas isn't constantly secreting insulin so you stop getting big insulin surges. The keto diet may also benefit some people suffering from migraines,[10] and it may help control seizures in some people with epilepsy who have not responded well to medication.[11] Experts are also finding that the brain functions better when it runs off fat than carbohydrates. "If you power your brain with fat, it's going to work better," Dr. David Perlmutter told us. "You're going to feel generally more energetic when you reduce what many people think is their best source of energy, sugar."[12]

Now for the flip. Some people feel worse on a keto diet. If you're used to a high-carb diet, then it'll take some time for your body to adjust. We hear a lot about "keto flu." This happens when your body is detoxing from the sugar it's used to eating. You may feel really uncomfortable while this happens.

There's also a phenomenon where the sugar-loving bacteria and yeast in the gut start to starve, and we can get a "die off" reaction that makes us feel feverish and generally crappy. You have to ride this out.

Keto and other low-carb diets limit carbs, so there's potential for insomnia and exhaustion too. Plus, modern-day fat is loaded with chemicals. By upping your fat intake on the keto diet, you could unintentionally be upping the chemicals in your body. If you're fat-loading, you're also eating a lot of pesticides, herbicides, and burnt plastic residue. Hello, cancer. Hello, exhaustion.

All of that said, keto can work as long as your body is optimized to do it properly. Your body needs to have the right enzymes to metabolize it and get it into the cells so your mitochondria can do their thing. But if your body can't digest and metabolize the fat right, you're in for a world of pain. Think looser, foul-smelling stools that come on out of nowhere and make you dash for the nearest bathroom. Not fun.

We won't tell you, yea or nay, to keto. Just weigh the pros and cons accordingly. If you do decide to try the keto way, if your budget allows, opt for organic, grass-fed, humanely raised meat.

Calorie Counting

Some nutritionists say to ditch the restrictions on calories. Others suggest counting them is a good thing. Which is it? To count or not to count?

At the end of the day, the logic of "calories in versus calories out" isn't wrong—it's simply not the full picture. If you count your calories but pay no attention to what *comprises* these calories, you're going to run into some serious problems.

Let's say you're on a 1,500-calorie restriction. You eat a donut and drink a latte for breakfast—that's 300 calories. You eat one of those packaged "health" bars for lunch—that's 200 calories. You eat a steak dinner and have two glasses of wine—that's 1,000 calories. Sure, you're right on the money, but you've missed the mark entirely for getting enough fiber, potassium, magnesium, B vitamins, vitamin A, K, or C—you haven't given your body very much nutrition at all. You've given it some protein and some sugar, and that's about it.

If you head for calorie counting, just make sure you're getting the proper nutrition.

Fasting

Flip history's pages and you'll see that some form of fasting has always been with us. Buddhists, Taoists, Hindus, Sikhs, Christians, Jews, Muslims—just about everyone knew the benefits of fasting and instilled this practice into their rituals. Check out the most popular health and nutrition blogs, and everyone's talking about fasting these days.

There are different types of fasts, and some of them are definitely better than others.

1. **Time-Restricted Eating.** This is when you give yourself a window of time to eat. Most of us live like this all the time—we don't eat between, say, 8 P.M. and 6 A.M. It's called "break-fast" for a reason. We call it fasting when we make that window a little larger, say between 6 P.M. and 6 A.M. That is a 12-hour fast. Some people work up to 14- or 16-hour fasts.

2. **Intermittent Fasting.** This is when you fast for a period of time. Perhaps you don't eat on Mondays. Perhaps you do a 3-day fast once a month. But the important part is taking a break in between, and not doing it over a long period of time.

3. **Long-Term Water Fasting.** This is a fast where you either subsist off just water, a light broth, or no food or water, and you do it for a longer period of time—the average is 10 days. These are intense fasts that many experts suggest should only be done under medical supervision.

People all over the world weren't wrong for all of those centuries —fasting has its benefits. Research shows it can improve metabolic health, blood sugar levels, mental clarity, and focus. Fasting also is like spring cleaning in your body. It helps stimulate *autophagy*, which is a cellular cleanup process. It goes in and cleans up the cellular material that's not working, including mutated cells that can later turn into cancer.

Fasting also does the same thing with your mitochondria, helping to stimulate a process called *mitophagy*, where your mitochondria get repaired or recycled so new, stronger ones are created.

If these benefits weren't enough, fasting can also help retrain and rewire your metabolic flexibility. When we are metabolically flexible, then it's easier for us to switch between the different fuel sources. It can even help some people induce mild ketosis where your body burns fat as fuel instead of the sugar from carbs.

These are great outcomes for sure, but there is a dark side to the practice. Fasting is not for everyone. If you have anxiety, hormone imbalances like thyroid problems, issues with sleep, or limbic system challenges (your limbic system handles your emotions, memories, and stimulation/arousal), then you're going to want to skip fasting. It can be really unsettling and bring up harsh emotional content. At the very least, make sure you have a good team of doctors and therapists in your corner if you insist on riding out to meet these dragons.

Also, if you've pounded carbs and sugars for most of your life, then you probably won't have the metabolic flexibility to switch from burning carbs to fat immediately. And if your energy is wrecked already, like you're barely able to drag yourself from bed, then forget it. Exhaustion and fasting are like mustard and peanut butter—they don't go. Your body is way too stressed and too depleted to take the strain. Fasting will make you more exhausted.

Once your energy has rebounded, then you can try playing around with fasting. When you do, start small. Recent research has found that the typical Westerner eats about 10 times per day over a total of 14–15 hours.[13] That's like the entire time you're awake.

If this sounds like a day in your life, take it easy with fasting. You're going to have to build and ease into the practice slowly. Experiment with longer breaks between meals. If your eating window is 14–16 hours, then gradually close it. Try eating for only 10–12 hours. Push back your breakfast so you eat from 9 A.M.–7 P.M. Do that a couple of times a week for a few weeks, and then close the window again. Try going from 10 A.M.–7 P.M., then 11 A.M.–7 P.M.

A restricted window during which you don't restrict your calories and don't miss any nutrients will give you most of the benefits of fasting, without much of the downside.

As your body gets accustomed to it, then you can start to play with more time-restricted feeding like six- or seven-hour feeding windows for a couple of days a week. Eventually you may build up to a 24- or 36-hour fast. If you're heading in that direction, you should consult a doctor, and definitely pay attention to how your body is responding to fasting.

When you bring fasting into your regimen, make sure your activity levels are balanced appropriately too. Don't try running marathons while fasting, and don't mistake it as a long-term strategy. Fasting is a great tool to occasionally throw into the mix to help boost energy and lose weight.

Energy Remedy #4:
Create a Healthy Relationship with Good Carbs

Not all carbs are bad. Squash, carrots, green beans, sweet potatoes, yams, fruit (unjuiced, and particularly berries), zucchini—these are all carbs. Eat them.

Where you really want to be cautious is with wheat. Just because something says "whole wheat" and is brown instead of white doesn't mean it's good for you. You might remember seeing something called "enriched flour" on the ingredients list. That means it's taken the nutrients *away*.

You want to go for 100 percent whole wheat, multigrain, fiber-rich breads. Even then, you might want to be a little cautious, because of the gluten factor. Avoiding gluten is another one of those things that often gets called a fad.

Also, part of the digestive process occurs in the gallbladder and pancreas. The gallbladder secretes bile, and the pancreas secretes enzymes, all of which we need to keep our energy system going. The gallbladder and pancreas know they need to get to work when they receive a signal from a hormone called cholecystokinin (CCK). Without CCK, we can't get the job done.

When gluten comes along, it inhibits the secretion of CCK. This leads to a reduction in enzyme function and more undigested food in the intestinal tract. This breakdown in the process can lead to nutrient deficiencies, infections in the intestinal tract, and more damage to the gut lining. What are the primary symptoms with nutrient deficiencies and gut inflammation? Exhaustion! And mind you, this can happen to *everybody*, not just people with celiac disease or gluten sensitivities.

There's something to be said for taking gluten out of your diet, but we admit, that can be hard to do. And sometimes, you just need some bread, dammit. The key is moderation. It's simple, we know. There's nothing exciting about it, but there's a lot of truth to it. If you're going to eat wheat products, including pasta and bread, take it easy. Don't make it a staple of your diet every day. Watch your intake, and pay attention to how your body responds. For some people, moderation is too much, so experiment with eliminating it from your diet and see how you feel. Some of the functional medical experts we spoke with said over 50 percent of their patients report feeling more energized and better overall after removing gluten from their diets.

Don't be afraid of carbs. Just make sure they're *good* carbs. Here are some gluten-free carbs you shouldn't be afraid of:

- Certified gluten-free whole rolled oats or oatmeal
- Leafy greens like lettuce, arugula, kale, and spinach
- Cruciferous vegetables like broccoli, brussels sprouts, and cabbage
- Brown rice, quinoa, and buckwheat
- Fruit, including bananas, oranges, apples, pears, and, especially, berries
- Starchy vegetables like corn, sweet potatoes, yams, squash, green beans, and carrots

Some options that include gluten are:

- Cereals with whole rolled oats, all-bran, muesli, and oatmeal (just make sure it's not heavily sweetened)
- Multigrain, 100% whole wheat breads
- Grains like barley, rye, and farro

Energy Remedy #5: Bring the Sacred to the Profane

Food is sacred. It's where your energy has come from, is coming from, and will forever come from as long as you live. A creature— even a living, breathing plant—lays down its life for you every day, at every meal. Let's be grateful for that being that has gifted us with its life force.

Let us bring the sacred back to the profane, to celebrate and pay tribute. We're not saying you need to literally say "grace" before every meal. If you want to, have at it. But returning gratitude to your mealtime is about repatterning your relationship with the earth through food and deep appreciation.

We're saying, understand where your food came from, what it's doing for you, what it's done for your ancestors, and the purpose of it in your life. And be grateful for that. Food isn't just something you write off as necessary and you go about your day.

Let's stop labeling food as a protein, a fat, a carbohydrate. Let's stop intellectualizing and disconnecting from our food and the supply chain. Most of us no longer have to kill our food, but someone did.

Let us be grateful to the animal, or plant, that has died so we could live. Let's practice gratitude before each meal, whether that's saying a silent prayer of "thanks" or speaking it aloud.

If you want to take your gratitude practices a step further, then consider reflecting on the meaning of *your* life. What are you doing with the life force you've been granted? How are you spending the energy you've consumed? Why do you believe you deserve life more than another?

We admit, these are some pretty deep, tough questions. But when it comes to restoring your energy, the introspective work, meaning of your life, and how you spend your energy matters a lot. We've devoted an entire chapter to these deeper questions and meaning (Chapter 9). You don't have to do anything with these questions right now. Just being willing to ask them and reflect on your answers is enough.

These are all ways to start bringing the sacred back into your life. Just try it for a week, and you will be amazed at the little energy boost you will feel from a practice that costs you nothing, but rewards you with everything.

SUCCESS STORY

It took Katie a long time to realize this, but she was actually getting pretty terrible advice from her dietician and her trainer.

It's not that what they were saying was bad or wrong—it just wasn't right *for her.* Katie's body responded differently to calorie counting than most of the people her dietician worked with. That kind of careful portioning made her crave sweets and fats, because she felt deprived all the time—and so she ate them. Katie didn't even realize she was doing it; she thought, *Hey, I'm well within my assigned calories, so it's all good!*

But it wasn't. A donut hole in lieu of an entire salad makes for a pretty unhealthy diet. No wonder she was so exhausted.

Here's the thing that helped Katie realize what was going on: when she works with her clients as a stylist, she always focuses on what makes them *feel* good. Katie might think Rebecca looks fantastic in 4-inch heels, but if Rebecca's worried that she's going to fall over, she's not going to feel confident. Therefore, the heels don't work.

Katie knows this—it's what makes her such a great stylist. But she hadn't been applying it to herself. Just as her clients know best what clothes will work for them, Katie knows what makes her body feel good.

She quit counting her calories, and just focused on eating foods that made her body happy. This meant skipping the immediate happiness of fat and sugar, and instead focusing on foods that made her feel light and energized—like quinoa and cashews, or kale chips when she needed a snack. She didn't pay as much attention to quantities, so she didn't feel deprived—and eventually, the pounds dropped off. She looked great and she felt great.

PERSONAL CHALLENGE

For a week, eat a good breakfast, something that will energize you and show you some immediate, positive change. We're talking slow carbs and protein, so that could be sweet potato hash and an egg, or a Polizzi favorite, loaded oatmeal with nuts, hemp seeds, raisins, cinnamon, and a little local honey.

CHAPTER 3

The Gut and Immune System

Michael's a very successful small-business owner. His web design company has revenues north of $5 million, and he's got a staff of 20. He loves his job, but about two years ago, his productivity and motivation tanked. He gained weight, and he noticed that his stomach often "felt off." He had a lot of bloating, gas, and was very constipated, then he started feeling sick, like he had a nasty head cold. This was strange because Michael never got sick.

Michael had seen five doctors and one therapist trying to get to the bottom of his exhaustion. He was desperate to get his mojo back. It wasn't just that the business was suffering. His wife was about to have their first baby, and he was in no shape to cope with that exhausting reality.

One doctor said his vitamin D levels were too low, so Michael was put on a supplement. Another doctor told him to go gluten-free, while another doctor told him to try a high-protein, low-carb diet, filled with lots of red meat and bacon. Then Michael switched to eating more vegetables, lean meats, fresh fruits, and some grains.

None of his diets made any difference. Michael was still sluggish, still gaining weight, still digestively "off," and his immune system was still acting up. In the last six months, he had two bouts of a nasty stomach flu, battled bronchitis, and kept cycling through terrible head colds.

He was burning out. His body was breaking down, and none of the experts seemed to know how to help him. Michael didn't know what to do or which doctor to see, and he was scared.

THE PROBLEM

You can eat the healthiest and cleanest diet on the planet, but if you can't digest your food and if your gut is inflamed, you're toast.

It's depressing, but true. Millions of us have gone to the trouble of cutting out sugar and processed foods, eating largely organic, whole ones. We've created pretty balanced diets filled with healthy macronutrients, and we're getting our vitamins and minerals. Yet our energy levels still suck. We feel terrible, and we have no idea why.

We go and see our general practitioner, and they have no answers for us either. In fact, most Western doctors will dismiss how we feel if there's nothing to see on our basic labs—a pretentious and dangerous reality many of us have experienced.

It's all too easy to start second-guessing, right? We figure, so what if our stomach hurts after a meal? What's the problem if we have to suddenly run for the bathroom? Who cares if we don't poop for three days—we've always been constipated? What's wrong with needing to lie down and take a nap after lunch?

We brush off weird or unexplainable GI issues as no big deal—but they are.

Our bodies communicate with us all the time, sending us subtle signals. GI issues are one of the ways our bodies speak to us, telling us something has gone off the rails. It's just that we've become extremely talented at ignoring or dismissing these messages.

Our culture doesn't teach us how to listen to the wisdom of our bodies. In fact, the notion of letting our senses explore every part of ourselves is bluntly discouraged by many of the world's major religions. (As children of two of the biggies, Islam and Catholicism, we had front-row seats growing up.)

But you have this ability.

It starts with learning how to recognize the subtle sensations your body gives to you in response to your lifestyle choices, especially with what you're eating and drinking.

Foods and beverages should make you feel energized, happy, and motivated because you just transformed what you consumed into energy. If after a meal you feel otherwise, then you have a problem. You have to start questioning and paying attention to what you're eating, how it's making you feel, and adjust accordingly.

You know your body better than anyone else (including us!). You know which foods your body thrives on, and which ones just don't support you.

We're here to help you learn to tap into these natural instincts, to return to your core and center, and to rediscover what foods work best for you and your energy. We want you to trust your body and live by what it's telling you.

Now, we definitely get that it's hard. When every food you eat seems to send your stomach lurching, twisting, and bellowing, it's difficult to hear what it actually needs.

When your body can't digest and use food in the way that it ought to, most of the time that's because your gut is inflamed and your immune system is off. If you're at the point Michael reached, your gut is basically on fire, and *nothing* works for it. We can help you put out the flames. We'll walk you through some of the possible causes like having imbalanced gut bacteria, low stomach acid, food intolerances or food allergies or leaky gut, and issues with your mitochondria.

As you read, have faith. It can be frustrating and take some time to heal GI issues, but you can heal your gut, and when you do, you'll feel better and your energy levels will be higher.

Be determined and patient. Lunch should be a treat, not a punishment.

THE ENERGY DRAINS

Energy Drain #1: Your Microbiome Has Been Invaded

You can't see them, but your body is home to an entire civilization, where trillions of organisms—friendly bacteria, fungi, and viruses—live. These bacteria outnumber your cells 10 to 1,[1] and most of them live inside your gut in what we call the *microbiome.*

These are the good guys. You need them to survive, and they need you too. These friendly bacteria help digest your food, regulate your immune system, and produce important vitamins such as B vitamins (thiamine, riboflavin, and biotin), amino acids like tryptophan and phenylalanine (needed for a stable mental state), and vitamin K, which you need for blood clotting.[2]

These good bacteria also fight off the bad bacteria, which can lead to autoimmune diseases or other illnesses.

When your gut bacteria are properly balanced, your microbiome is healthy and you're filled with energy. But when your gut bacteria become unbalanced, all hell gets unleashed. Everyone has some bad bacteria inside their microbiome, but when the good bacteria get outnumbered, the bad guys will colonize and take control.

When that happens, your good bacteria can't complete their jobs like helping you digest your food, bolstering your immune system, and keeping your body healthy and happy. End result? You're drained and exhausted.

How did the bad bacteria gain control?

Our story begins millions of years ago, when our friendly bacteria started to co-evolve with us. Back when our ancestors roamed the land, they ate mostly high-fiber vegetables—think gnarly carrots that had to work really hard to grow through soil and minerals. Our ancestors would yank out that carrot, brush off a bit of dirt, and chow down. They were eating the bacteria from the dirt and consuming lots of nutrients and fiber from the carrot.

Some of that fiber, they couldn't digest, so it was given to the friendly bacteria like a sacrificial offering. The friendly bacteria chewed it right up, feasting, growing stronger, and multiplying their population. In turn, they worked hard helping B.C. *Homo sapiens* to better digest their food, create more vitamins, and stave off any troublemaking bad bacteria they might ingest.

Way back when, our ancestors ate around 100 grams of fiber a day.[3] Today, most of us are eating *between 10–15 grams.*[4] It's recommended that women up to the age of 50 eat 25 grams per day, while those over 50 should eat 21 grams.[5] For men up to the age of 50, that number should be 38 grams, and for those over 50, that number drops to 30.[6]

And the food we're eating is nowhere near as powerful or healthy. When plants don't have to fight for their survival, they grow up weak. A blueberry growing on a scraggly bush on a mountainside is going to be way more nourishing than its big fat hothouse cousin.

What makes the difference? That blueberry shrub on the mountainside faced tons of insects, got less water, and had to live through cold, harsh winters. The best, most nutrient-rich blueberries on that bush had to fend for themselves, and they became more resilient and stronger in the process. When you eat those blueberries, you're taking in a stronger life force, better energy, and better nutrients.

But modern agricultural practices have nuked the soil and the plants, and killed off all the bugs. By doing so, they've made plants lazy. Plants today have less nutritional value than they did just a generation ago.

This is compounded by the drastic increase in conventional use of antibiotics. These days, doctors prescribe antibiotics as if they were candy, oftentimes handing them out for illnesses that they are absolutely useless against. These antibiotics are killing off the good bacteria in our guts—and making the bad bacteria stronger.

Unfortunately, even if you're using these prescriptions responsibly, the reality is that you are still unknowingly ingesting antibiotics by eating nonorganic meats. Cows, pigs, and chickens are all routinely injected with antibiotics and other toxins. The idea here is to increase yield, to make animals that can survive in crowded, unhealthy conditions.

Add on the lack of stomach acid, and it means food goes undigested in the gut. Guess which bacteria absolutely pig-out on the rotting food? Yep, the bad bacteria.

Put all together, it causes our friendly bacteria to grow weaker and stop multiplying. This means they can't do their jobs breaking down food, making vitamins, and warding off the bad guys.

To make it worse—oh yes, this story gets worse—you've unknowingly been beefing up the bad guys. High-fiber diets have largely been replaced with high-sugar diets. Which bacteria do you think thrives on this?

You guessed it again: bad bacteria.

Sugar can lurk in lots of food and drinks. Those energy drinks you may be guzzling to keep you going during the day? They can contain anywhere between 26 and a whopping 83.5 grams of sugar per serving!

You have unwittingly aided and abetted the enemy. The bad bacteria have grown stronger. They have multiplied their troops. They have invaded your microbiome. They have colonized your gut, defeated and subdued the good guys, and are now lighting firestorms throughout your body.

When bad bacteria outnumber the good guys, you can get yeast or candida overgrowth, and parasites. You can get terrible indigestion, gas, bloating, diarrhea, or constipation. You can experience painful acid reflux. You can even get brain fog and mood changes.

And your energy levels will suck, since the good guys aren't there to break down your food into life-giving vitamins and minerals.

Energy Drain #2:
Your Immune System Is Trapped in an Endless War

Your immune system is your protection against foreign invaders. Think of it as your military designed to stand guard and keep your body safe against bad bacteria, viruses, undigested food particles, and anything that shows up where it doesn't belong. About 70 percent of that immune system lives in your gut, where it's known as the gut-associated lymphoid tissue, or GALT.

If your gut isn't functioning well, your immune system won't either. That means serious trouble for you and your energy levels.

Your immune system and the good bacteria are on the same side. They have a two-way communication. The good bacteria are found in the gut lining, which is basically a tube from your mouth to your anus. (We know that's a lovely image. You're welcome.)

This tube is like purgatory. It's a halfway house between what's considered inside and outside your body. Just because you swallowed some food doesn't mean it's actually in your body. It has to cross over the gut lining first. Somewhere between the small and the large intestine, the good bacteria, stomach acids, and enzymes will break down the food into vitamins, minerals, and macronutrients.

Once the food breaks down into small enough molecules, it passes through your gut lining—now it's in your body and ready to be delivered via your bloodstream to all your organs, muscles, and tissues. Whatever doesn't break down gets pooped out.

As this digestive process happens, your immune system stands watch, constantly asking, "Is this food friend or foe?"

If it's a friend, the food passes into the bloodstream peacefully. If it's a foe, it's time for war.

Part of the exhaustion equation comes from all the crap food that your immune system doesn't recognize. You're tossing down Cheetos coated with Sunset Yellow FCF or guzzling energy drinks loaded with Blue No. 1, and your immune system is like, "What the hell is this? It ain't food. Destroy it!"

If the bad bacteria, viruses, fungi, and parasites are outnumbering the good guys—or get outside the gut lining and into your bloodstream—your immune system will also kick into high gear, charging in to protect its turf.

To eliminate a threat, the immune system first sends scout cells called *macrophages* to seek out the intruder. Once found, the scouts chew 'em up to subdue the enemy, and then call in the soldier cells, the natural-born killer *T cells*, to come in and finish off the invader.

Sometimes finding the invader proves difficult. Your body is a big place. Your immune system calls in reinforcements—that would be your *B cells*, which make *antibodies* that bind to the invader, marking them for elimination, so your T cells can swoop in and take them out.

This is the war for your health and well-being, and it is being waged every minute of every hour of every day, for your entire life. Your immune system is doing exactly what it was designed to do.

But all of this warfare causes a lot of inflammation, and if you're constantly inflamed because your immune system is always at DEF-CON 3 or lower, you'll start having some serious side effects, including bloating, indigestion, heartburn, diarrhea, and constipation. You might experience brain fog, memory loss, insomnia, and even more exhaustion.

You feel like shit because the bad bacteria have colonized your gut, and you feel like shit because your body's trying to take out the bad guys. It's like kickboxing with a broken leg.

This is a very bad thing. Science has begun to find that the common underpinning to almost every modern-day disease—diabetes, heart disease, obesity, thyroid problems, Crohn's, achy joints, skin issues like eczema, and even cancer—is inflammation.

If your immune system is constantly having to defend against the unhealthy food, bad bacteria, and viruses, then it will get overloaded really fast and start to go haywire. Most of the functional medicine doctors we spoke with believe that autoimmune diseases begin in the gut—so now you're looking at issues like rheumatoid arthritis, lupus, irritable bowel syndrome, psoriasis, Hashimoto's, and more. Your immune system can no longer tell friend from foe.

Your immune system can go haywire even when you eat seemingly healthy foods. "When you have a person who's usually eating fast food, and the same food every day, or the same salad with their four vegetables and the ones they don't like are off, and they don't even have a variety of plants, they will lose the microbiome diversity and food tolerance," said Dr. Datis Kharrazian, a Harvard Medical School–trained and award-winning clinical research scientist, academic professor, and world-renowned functional medicine health care provider. "Even though they think they're eating healthy, they get systemic inflammation, and that can disrupt energy metabolism, and now they're fatigued."[7]

There is a chaotic war between the food you're eating and your immune system raging inside your body, often without you realizing it. All you know is you're beyond tired and feel like crap.

Energy Drain #3: Your Stomach Acid Has Disappeared

Your metabolism starts in your gut. If your gut health isn't in good shape, it doesn't matter what you eat or drink—you're not going to absorb the micronutrients or the macronutrients.

No nutrients? No energy.

This is the sad state many people find themselves stuck in. They eat, but they can't digest their food because they don't have enough stomach acid. To digest your food, especially protein, you need a lot of hydrochloric acid. Hydrochloric acid (we'll call it *stomach acid* from here on) plays a key role in breaking your food into small molecules that your mitochondria will use to create ATP.

Unfortunately, many Americans don't produce enough stomach acid to properly break down their food. Chronic stress, eating too quickly, eating too much sugar, or vitamin deficiencies—particularly zinc or B vitamins—are among the causes of low stomach acid. When you don't have enough stomach acid, it means your body isn't breaking down that grilled chicken or T-bone steak.

When you don't produce enough stomach acid, and you can't break down the food, it just hangs out in your gut, rotting. You end up with nasty acidic by-products that can lead to gastroesophageal reflux disease (GERD), causing reflux, indigestion, and other downstream issues.

You really don't feel well when this happens, so you head to your general practitioner, and what's your doc's solution? He gives you proton pump inhibitors or other antacids, which, sure, they neutralize the acids and make you feel better for a little while, but they really just exacerbate the overall problem. Most people with this issue have *more* hydrochloric acid, not less.

But the antacid medications your doctor put you on bring your pH to around 5.0 in a matter of weeks, which is more like (technically less than) table vinegar. All that does is marinate your protein-rich food, rather than digesting it. The normal acid level in the stomach should be around 1.7 to 1.9—this is closer to battery acid. That's really acidic, but your stomach lining has a special protective substance that prevents it from dissolving.

Now, producing stomach acid in the first place requires *a ton* of energy (ATP). In fact, it's one of the most energy-dependent reactions in the body. If you're exhausted, you likely don't have enough ATP, and if you don't have enough ATP, then you also don't have enough stomach acid to break down your food to make more ATP.

Cue the terrible, vicious spiral that becomes exhaustion.

If you don't have the stomach acid you need to break down your food to extract the energy you need, you're screwed. And very quickly, that undigested food starts to wreak mayhem and madness throughout your system.

Energy Drain #4: You're Battling Undigested Food Molecules and Leaky Gut

This immune response and all that inflammation we just described doesn't just happen when we eat shit food. It can happen with the healthy stuff too. If you don't have enough stomach acid or enzymes to break down your food, or if you don't have the good bacteria helping you digest, then your immune system can start to recognize *any* food as an enemy.

Welcome to the world of food sensitivities and allergies. *Food sensitivities or food intolerances* happen when you can't digest your food. They often cause gas, bloating, diarrhea, and other GI issues. Food allergies are slightly different and occur when our immune system overreacts. They can be life threatening. Foods that often cause allergic reactions in people include peanuts, cow's milk, soy, shellfish, or wheat.

It's no secret that gluten, dairy, grains, soy, and legumes tend to cause the most inflammation. These foods are just harder for your gut to break down. But what many people don't realize is that they could eat the healthiest food in the world—lean meats and loads of vegetables—and their immune systems would still go on the offensive. This was part of Michael's problem. He was eating healthy foods like turkey and chicken and lots of fresh vegetables, but he couldn't digest them, so his immune system was on high alert.

We'll add one more layer to this complicated web of misery: leaky gut.

When you don't have enough stomach acid to properly digest your food, then your gut lining can begin to deteriorate, and gaps can form. If you have gaps in your stomach lining, then bad bacteria, toxins, and undigested food particles can sneak through and get into your bloodstream.

Say you munched on a Krispy Kreme donut during your morning meeting. Your body can't digest it all the way, so you're left with a gluten molecule that floats through a gap in your stomach lining and right into your bloodstream.

It's not supposed to be there, so your immune system immediately responds. As we described earlier, part of our defense is to create antibodies that will bind to the invader, so your killer cells can attack and destroy.

It sounds good in theory. But the problem is that your body has now learned to interpret the gluten molecule as a foe. Anytime you eat gluten now, your body attacks, and when your body attacks, you get inflammation. You may feel bloated, gassy, have bowel problems, get indigestion, feel nauseous, or experience stomach pains. You'll also probably be super tired because of the resulting sugar crash.

We used a donut as our test subject, but this can happen with *anything* you eat. That hardboiled egg didn't digest all the way and it floats through your gut lining? Uh-oh, off your immune system races to destroy. Same with dairy, soy, corn, egg, nuts—pick your poison. These are some of the more commonly reactive foods.

If you're experiencing this, you probably have no idea that it's going on. It's not like we can see the holes in our gut lining.

And, we have to tell you, while leaky gut is a proven issue in the body and a cause of disease, modern medicine doesn't recognize it as a thing.

You're probably sitting there going, "Could I be allergic to the foods I eat?" Well, maybe. Not in the "you need a damn EpiPen or you'll go into anaphylactic shock and possibly die" sort of allergic way—more in the "this damn mosquito bite is bugging the shit out of me" way.

For instance, if you eat a steak and have gas, that's a sign: Don't eat it. You probably have some food intolerance happening because you're not properly digesting your food.

But if on the other hand you take a bite of shrimp and your face starts swelling, you're probably allergic and need to take that out of your diet. Nick loves eating cheese. It is one of his favorite foods—but it causes some serious side effects like breaking out in a cold sweat and face swelling. Turns out, he has a dairy allergy. For years, he shrugged it off and never paid much attention to the sweating and swelling. Actually, he figured it was something that happened to everyone.

Once he took dairy out of his diet, he didn't have those strange ailments. Sure, he misses cheese, but he feels better after he eats. He has more energy and doesn't have weird reactions. Food allergies can have some very serious, life-threatening effects, so don't mess around.

Your gut is the front line in turning food into energy. If you're eating foods that your body is having an immune response to, then you're screwed. You aren't creating energy from your food—you're actually using what little energy you have left to attack what you just ate.

Let's look at two scenarios. In Scenario One, you've got a leaky gut. Your undigested food molecules are floating through your gut lining to do battle with your immune system. In Scenario Two, you don't have enough good bacteria, stomach acid, or enzymes to break down your food, so it's just hanging around in your gut, doing battle with your immune system (and expanding the population of your bad bacteria too).

In either scenario, you're set up for exhaustion.

Energy Drain #5:
Your Mitochondrial Warriors Are Down

In the last chapter, we talked about how your mitochondria live inside your cells, making energy (ATP). They also have another job—to defend your cells against threats. They can do only one job at a time.

Your mitochondria aren't just living isolated lives inside your cells either. Modern science is just learning about the intricate communication happening between our friendly gut bacteria *and* our mitochondria. Turns out, they're talking to each other all the time, telling each other if everything's okay in the neighborhood or if there's a bad guy hanging on the corner.

When you have some bad bacteria in the gut or a stray undigested food particle floating outside your gut lining, the good bacteria will tell your mitochondria to mount up and defend your cells against the invader. If your gut is clear, then the good bacteria let the mitochondria know they should stand down and just keep chugging to produce more energy.

This is the story of bacteria and mitochondria. It's happening in the background, and nobody completely understands it yet—but we do know that it's absolutely impacting our energy levels.

If your friendly gut bacteria are telling your mitochondria to shut off energy production and prepare to defend, then they're going to switch from being energy producers to defenders of the cellular realm. "The more that your mitochondria are picking up on those danger signals, the more it shuts down energy mode and turns on danger mode or defense mode," said Ari Whitten. "Fatigue is a problem of the mitochondria being switched too much into defense mode and taken out of energy mode."[8]

Part of the exhaustion challenge is that your mitochondria have been kept armed and ready for far too much of the time, and so they simply aren't able to produce enough energy. Our mitochondria and friendly gut bacteria have been hanging together for millions of years and, frankly, we're the dumb host stuck in the middle. The communication between them, the genetic expression that cues from there, and the subsequent energy production are the subjects of some incredible research happening right now. It's exciting and earth-shattering.

We're learning more daily, but the moral of the story we currently understand is this: eat real food and nurture your microbiome. When you do that, your friendly gut bacteria will signal to your mitochondria that all is well and will tell them, "Keep making energy for this creature; it's a good bet."

Personal Quest (Pedram)

For years, I had dark circles under my eyes. I figured it was some Middle Eastern genetic thing since my parents are from Iran. But it turns out that every time I eat dairy or drink alcohol, or do one of the other things that causes my immune system to go haywire, my blood vessels widen, the blood pools under my eyes, and I get dark circles.

It's not a huge deal, right? I mean, I have to go on TV sometimes, but when I've got dark circles, they make me put makeup on—which makes me feel super masculine. But I'm not bleeding or writhing around on the floor or anything. It's minor.

Sometimes I just say the hell with it. It's an immunological issue, and so it's within my control. I've got kids, and sometimes I've got to do things that maybe I shouldn't for the sake of convenience and simplicity. Sometimes I don't ask what's in the pumpkin pie at Thanksgiving, or I have that glass of red wine. I'll pay for it later, but because it *is* minor, I have the luxury of doing that.

But here's the thing: if I eat those foods or drink too much alcohol too often, I experience more than just dark circles. My symptoms get worse, and I'll reach a point where I'll need to either sleep for a month and fix my immune system, or I'll end up writhing around on the floor with terrible GI issues. If I hit that point, then no more pumpkin pie for me, for a very long time.

It's about choice and paying attention to what we're eating and how we're feeling after.

TESTS

The first thing you need to fix your gut issues is more information. There are a slew of tests that functional medical practitioners use to unlock the mysteries of your gut. Tests and jargon can seem confusing, so we're giving you the nuts and bolts on some of the most popular examinations. Use this information to empower you to ask questions and be your own advocate.

Amino Acid/Enzyme Test

You may have low amino acid levels, including histidine, an amino acid needed to make gastric acid. Amino acid and mineral insufficiencies are clues to tell you that you may be low in gastric acid, as stomach acid is needed to digest these nutrients from your food. Try fecal elastase-1, which is a test that will give a clue if your pancreatic enzymes are being secreted (you can ask your general practitioner about this).

Lipase/Bile Test

If you have fat in your stool, you're likely missing lipase or bile or both. Steatocrit, or fecal fat, analysis will measure the fat content of your stool.

Food Sensitivity

A food sensitivity test will show which foods nourish your body, and which ones cause you inflammation.

Organic Acids

Based on urine samples, medical professionals can discover how your physiology is functioning. They can see how well your mitochondria turn fats, carbohydrates, and proteins into ATP. They can also see if you have B-vitamin deficiencies or bacterial or fungal imbalances in your gut. Some good sources for this test are Organix from Genova Diagnostics and the Great Plains Laboratory Organic Acids Test (otherwise known as the GPL OAT).

Stool Test

This shows how well you're digesting the fats and proteins from your food. It'll show if bad bacteria have taken over, or if there are parasites compromising your immune system. Take a look at Viome, GI Effects, GI MAP, or the CDSA (the comprehensive digestive stool analysis).

DIY Digestion Quiz

How can you tell if you're not metabolizing your food correctly? Here are three easy questions to help you identify what macronutrient you may have trouble digesting.

Proteins: Do you have a heavy feeling in your body, like food is not moving, particularly after consuming any of the following?

    a. Nuts

    b. Meats

    c. Other sources of protein

If proteins are sitting in your gut like a lead weight, this may mean you are lacking the acid to digest them.

Carbohydrates: After eating, do you experience any of the following?

    a. Gas

    b. Nausea

    c. Burping

    d. Bloating

    e. Gooey soft-serve poops

If you answered yes to any of the above, you may have an issue with carbohydrate digestion.

Fats: When you poop, do you experience any of the following?

    a. Floating stools

    b. Lighter colored stools

    c. Foul-smelling stools (Yes, shit always stinks. But sometimes it stinks more than other times.)

If you answered yes to any of the above, it could mean you're having trouble digesting fat.

THE ENERGY REMEDIES

Energy Remedy #1: Bring Back the Good Bacteria

Simplicity is your friend when it comes to bringing back your good bacteria. There's no one-and-done remedy here, but there are a few adjustments you can make to your diet to bolster your troops.

Eat More Fiber

Your friendly bacteria love anything that's high in fiber and low in sugar. We're talking whole grains, leafy greens, quinoa, all of those good complex carbohydrates that we mentioned in Chapter 2. Preferably organic foods too, which are lower in pesticides and higher in the good bacteria.

Cut Back on Simple Carbs and Sugar

If you haven't already, start cutting back on your simple carbohydrates like white breads, bagels, snack foods, even those gluten-free bars that come in wrappers. That's the stuff your bad bacteria and yeasts go crazy for.

Eat Probiotic and Prebiotic Foods

Want to give your friendly bacteria a population boost? Then add more *probiotics*—foods that contain friendly bacteria—to your diet. Fall in love with fermented foods like kimchee, sauerkraut, kombucha, apple cider vinegar, miso, tempeh, or yogurt—not the sugary stuff.

Now, probiotics are not the magical cure. They're great, but they're not the whole story. If you take in these probiotics, you need to support them with *prebiotics*. These are specialized plant fibers that support your friendly gut bacteria. You can get prebiotics in many complex carbohydrates like bananas, garlic, onions, green beans, berries, root vegetables, and leafy greens.

Do both in sufficient quantities, and your friendly bacteria will start reproducing and overwhelm all the bad guys.

Eat a Varied Diet Filled with Organic Produce and Humanely Raised Animal Protein

"The more diversity you have in the microbiome, the less reactive you are to food proteins and to the environment," said Dr. Datis Kharrazian.[9]

If you're someone who lives off eating the same foods for breakfast, lunch, and dinner, it's time to switch it up. You want diversity in your microbiome, so you need to eat diverse foods. You're an interesting person. Eat interesting food.

And focus on incorporating lots of whole, unprocessed, unrefined foods that nourish your body and restore your energy. Choose organic produce when your bank account allows. Not only is it free of chemicals and pesticides that may harm you and your gut microbes, but it's proven to have more vitamins and minerals than nonorganic produce. It's also better for the environment.

When you can, choose grass-fed meat—humanely raised. What animals eat, we eat. Choose wisely.

Energy Remedy #2: Opt for an Anti-Inflammatory Diet

Food can either work with you or against you. Certain foods like gluten, grains, sugar, yeast, dairy, and soy can trigger an inflammatory response in many people. When you're living day after day with an inflamed gut, then you have to calm it down.

Many people have found healing and renewed energy by adopting an anti-inflammatory elimination diet. It's exactly what it says, and it's nothing new. You remove the foods that are highly inflammatory, giving your gut a chance to recover. For many people, they go off gluten, dairy, grains, soy, and sugar—yes, all of them, all at once.

When you get the inflammation in your gut down, all your organs function better. Your friendly bacteria start multiplying and strengthening. You start feeling clearheaded and energetic.

Some people even lose weight. Skin conditions like adult acne, eczema, and psoriasis can also improve. Others report strange pains in places like behind the ear, or a bulge in the back, disappear along with the inflammation.

The diet is simple, but it does take discipline. You have to commit to eliminating these foods entirely for *at least four weeks*. Then you start reintroducing a food every three days and tracking how your body responds. Remember, listen to your body. It won't lie to you. If you eat something and you react with gas, indigestion, or a strange stitch in your side, you'll know it's caused by the reintroduced food.

If a month seems too long, then try this: go caveman. Just eat natural foods, vegetables, fruits, and lean meats. Nothing processed. No sugar. And ditch the grains. Try it for two weeks. If you feel better, then you know your body's reacting to some food.

Just like the elimination diet, you can start to add foods back one at a time every few days to measure your response. If it turns out you don't have a problem with soy, great! But if gluten makes your gut unhappy, then you know what you need to do.

There is so much information that you can discover without spending thousands on tests. This is something you can do on your own, from your own home, and all it takes is a little pre-meal planning and a journal.

The elimination diet is a phenomenal training tool that will help you learn to listen and understand your body's messages. It's always talking to you, and it will tell you what foods it needs, how much it needs, and when. Think of this as the master reset button that can help you rediscover the foods you can eat without getting inflamed. From there, you can slowly branch out.

You may find that dairy, especially milk or cheese from a cow, doesn't settle with you. But goat cheese may be fine for you. You may also surprise yourself. Once you bump up your good bacteria, you might be able to enjoy an even more diverse diet—including the occasional splurge.

Energy Remedy #3: Get That Gastric Acid Flowing

If you're low on stomach acid, eating will be a pain—literally. We've got to change that, and here are a few tips to up your stomach acid production.

Get Off the Antacids

Studies have shown that antacids can increase the risk of food allergies[10] and that someone on antacid medication is twice as likely to be prescribed anti-allergy medication too.[11] This shows that there could be a link between antacid medications and an increase in immune system reactions.

The takeaway here: if you're on antacids, talk with your doctor about getting off them. No more proton pump inhibitors, no more Prilosec—we're even giving over-the-counter antacids the side-eye. Just beware, there will be a rebound period after going off these medications that can make you feel miserable for the first four to seven days. If this is the case, just eat some food. Good, whole foods are best, but the idea here is to give the acid something to do other than eat you.

Eat Slowly and Chew Your Food

Eating slowly and chewing wasn't just something your mom told you as a kid so you wouldn't choke. Turns out, when we eat and chew our food, it activates our gastric acid production. Tasting your food instead of sucking it up like a vacuum will signal to your brain to tell your digestive organs what type of macronutrient needs breaking down.

Chewing is so important. If you can't break macro molecules down to micro pieces, you'll never even get to the tiny particles you need to make ATP. When you chew your food really well, it increases the surface area of the food, which gives your enzymes and gastric acid more to work with. A 2009 study found that chewing your almonds 25 times versus 10 times significantly increases the energy the subjects got from them.[12]

Get Relaxed

When we're relaxed, it ramps up our gastric acid production. How do we relax while we eat? Well, first off, shut off your phone. Put it on airplane mode and stick it in another room. Don't have the news playing in the background. Shut off the television, radio, or that podcast. Listen to peaceful music, or if you're on your lunch break, try eating outside or in the cafeteria. Just don't eat at your desk in front of your computer.

Pay attention to what you're eating. Think about it. What does it taste like? What is the texture? Look at what's on your plate. Take some deep breaths before you take a bite. Smell your food. All of these seemingly small acts will help to activate your parasympathetic nervous system—this is your relaxed state.

Eat More Bitters

A meal starts with taste. We have five flavors to work with: salt, umami, sweet, sour . . . and bitter. The first four have one series of taste buds, but bitter has 26 different classes of taste buds.

Why do we have this? Because bitter-tasting foods like alkaloids and terpenes *can kill you.* Your body needs to know if you're eating something poisonous, so it's dedicated a lot of sensors to figuring that out.

Of course, not all bitter things are poisonous. Coffee, dark chocolate, bitter greens, roots, and more are all delicious, but their bitter flavor tells your digestive system to get into high gear just in case this turns out to be a poison. It does this in an efficient, healthy way—this isn't your digestive system overworked; it's your digestive system working how it's supposed to.

Energy Remedy #4: Heal Your Gut Lining

Feeding the good gut bacteria and the elimination diet can help a lot of people restore energy quickly. But if you've got leaky gut, then it doesn't matter what you eat—anything could trigger your immune system and inflammation. If that's the case for you, it's time to heal that lining first. All it takes are the right nutrients, and those gaps in the gut lining can close.

Butyrate is a kind of fatty acid that helps your gut. It helps control the growth of the cells lining your gut. When you have adequate butyrate, your gut lining has less permeability and less inflammation in general. You can get butyrate by eating more fiber. It's also found in butter and full-fat dairy products (assuming you can tolerate those foods).

Glutamine is an amino acid that the cells in your gut lining can use to heal. You can get glutamine from eating animal protein, as well as cabbage and beans. It's also available as a supplement. By increasing your glutamine intake, your stomach lining will start to heal. And, bonus—glutamine is a precursor for certain neurotransmitters that cause sugar cravings, and cutting down those cravings will stop you from feeding the bad bacteria in your gut.

Energy Remedy #5: Get That Mitophagy Pumping

Want to support the communication between your good bacteria and your mitochondria? Then try eating more pomegranates, the fruit of the gods. Pomegranates (along with grapes, pecans, walnuts, and most berries) have ellagic acid, a powerful antioxidant. On its own, ellagic acid will treat inflammation, but when your good bacteria break down ellagic acid, it becomes a compound called *Urolithin A*.

Urolithin A is one of the most powerful promoters of *mitophagy*. This is the process where any mitochondria that are exhausted and aren't producing as much energy or defending the cell as well get repaired. If the damage or stress to the mitochondria is too great, they get cleaned out to make room for new, revitalized, ready-to-get-to-work mitochondria.

This is a natural process, and a much-needed one that keeps your mitochondria at peak performance.

Energy Remedy Bonus: Slurp That Bone Broth

Bone broth is enjoying its moment in the spotlight today. When you're having GI issues, adding bone broth to your diet can do wonders for healing your stomach. "Bone broth gives you an abundance of nutrition, and at the same time, it detoxifies you," explained Dr. Kellyann Petrucci, a New York City–based, board-certified naturopathic physician, certified nutrition consultant, and bone broth expert.[13]

As Dr. Petrucci told us, bone broth is low calorie and low carb, yet it's highly nutritious. That's partly because bone broth has something in it called *collagen*. Collagen is the glue that holds your body together and uplifts you. About 33 percent of your body is actually collagen. It's the most abundant protein in your body.

Bone broth is also a killer protein source that can build up your amino acids, so you can digest your food better. In Chinese medicine, bone broth has been used for thousands of years to support digestive health and to build up your blood supply. Just adding two cups of bone broth to your diet, say first thing in the morning, and even at your next 3 P.M. lull, can make a difference in your health and energy levels.

Bone broth is readily available in stores, but it's easy enough to make yourself. Start with about two pounds of bones (chicken, beef, whatever) and pour a gallon of water over them, along with two tablespoons of apple cider vinegar (the vinegar will help release the nutrients of the bones).

If you want, you can add vegetables like celery, carrots, onions, garlic, and various herbs and spices, which will make the broth even better for you. Bring the whole thing to a boil, and let it simmer for a long time.

What do we mean by a long time? Twenty-four hours for chicken, and forty-eight hours for beef. If any yuck floats to the top, skim it off and just let it keep cooking.

SOLUTION

Michael finally connected to a functional medical practitioner who tested him for food sensitivities. Lo and behold, there they were. He learned that his gut was inflamed, and his body was rejecting most of the foods he was eating.

He also had several nutrient deficiencies (not surprising, since he wasn't able to fully digest the food he was consuming). He had already been placed on a vitamin D supplement by a traditional doctor, but his functional medicine practitioner told him to go to the source—sunshine.

In people who do not digest fat well, vitamin D is hard to absorb. It requires fat to help the body process it, but Michael was rejecting the foods that would help him. On the other hand, the body is designed to get its vitamin D from the sun—that's how our ancestors got their doses. Michael was instructed to spend at least 30 minutes in the morning and afternoon under those natural rays—sans sunscreen, because the UV rays are where the good stuff is. Michael needed to be careful, since skin cancer is no picnic either, but this was an effective and natural way to get his body the nutrients it needs. (Check out the dminder app. It's free and will tell you how much sun you need in your area to get a good dose of vitamin D without burning your skin!)

His functional medicine practitioner also worked with him to create an anti-inflammatory nutrition plan for his body. He started by eliminating the foods that he was sensitive to, and instead eating leafy vegetables, fruits, nuts, and fatty fish. He was also put on anti-inflammatory supplements that were easy for his body to absorb, like alpha-lipoic acid, curcumin, and fish oil.

In just four weeks, Michael's energy levels rebounded. And when his vitamin D levels were checked, his numbers had skyrocketed for the first time in five years.

Doesn't sound all that difficult? It wasn't. It required some discipline, but after two years of chronic fatigue, Michael had no problem doing the work to get his gut working for him again.

PERSONAL CHALLENGE

Cut out the sugar for a week. Make a note of how you feel after each day. Are you gassy? How are your bowel movements? Do you feel tired? Do you feel bloated? Do you feel more energized?

One week, no sugar—you can do this.

CHAPTER 4

Exercise and Movement

Amy was 65 years old. She thought she was reasonably active—she worked in her garden, and she took her dog on walks. Sometimes she went on short hikes with her granddaughter.

But then one day, her friends from book group were talking about how little exercise they'd been getting. They were talking about their weight. They weren't talking about Amy specifically—her friends would never do that—but Amy felt self-conscious. Mary Ann was moaning about her weight and saying she needed to exercise more—but Amy knew for a fact that Mary Ann went to a Power Yoga class three times a week, and she looked *great*.

Amy took a sip of wine, and noticed the way her upper arms jiggled. She felt her hips spreading across the seat of her chair. "Maybe I'll come with you to yoga tomorrow," she told Mary Ann.

Amy did go to class, and at first it felt great. But the class just kept going . . . long past when Amy was tired. She became dizzy, and she wanted to rest, but she didn't want to be the only person sitting out the class. How humiliating it would be for Mary Ann to see her like that.

Her face turned red, and she was gasping for breath, but she pushed through. There were some movements she wasn't really ready for, and she fell. And the next day, she was so sore she could barely walk.

She couldn't face it again. And so, when Mary Ann asked her about coming to the next class, she said she was busy. Eventually, Mary Ann stopped asking.

Amy did want to lose weight. She knew she needed to be more active. But she didn't know where to start. She felt like a failure.

THE PROBLEM

For so many people, exercise is misery. But it doesn't have to be that way. In this chapter, we're going to help give you the boost you need to climb out from your pit of despair.

This chapter is all about transforming your relationship with exercise and movement, because let's face it, odds are, you're probably in a dysfunctional relationship with it. That's why we're peeling back some of the psychological and physical energy drains that are knocking you out from the game of life.

This isn't about showing you *how* to exercise. It's about inspiring you to *want* to make it a part of your life, to see it as one of the most fun and enjoyable, and down-right addicting ways to renew your life force—because it is.

For both of us, exercising and movement are a huge part of living and being in this world. It's how we get the juice to raise our families, to run businesses, to make films, to write books, and do the thousands of other things that make life worth living.

It's also one of the most important tools that all of us have to manage stress. When our ancestors encountered stress, it usually resulted in physical movement. Some ferocious animal or someone from another tribe chased them. They had to turn and fight or they kept running. A physical release went with that fight-or-flight response.

Fast forward to today, and most of our stress is internal. It's worrying about our kids, about money, about our government, about climate change, about the upcoming meeting with our bosses.

As a consequence, we now "sit and stew."

It's even more important now to bring intentional movement into your day. Exercise can counteract stress. "When we get physical exercise, it's like we're getting the benefits of the top-selling pharmaceutical drugs without any of the side effects," said Dr. Heidi Hanna, an expert in stress mastery and brain-based health and performance.[1]

Moving through the world is a part of being alive. If you're not moving, you're a dead animal. Yes, we said animal. We know, we don't like to consider ourselves animals, but if we could remind ourselves that we are part of the animal kingdom, we might remember and learn about life, its meaning, and our connection to Mother Nature.

The amazing thing with exercise and movement is that everyone can do it. Even if you're limited by disabilities or injuries, even if you're severely overweight, even if you're so exhausted that walking for five minutes seems too much, you can find *something* to do.

Stay curious in, and feel empowered to take control of, your life once more.

THE ENERGY DRAINS

Energy Drain #1: You've Bought into a False Narrative

Remember when we talked about how the world was broken and you nodded your head? Well, keep nodding, because we're going to deprogram all the toxicity that you've been force-fed around exercise, movement, and your image.

Hollywood, the ad industry, magazines, and the media have all told you to value how you look more than how you feel. Most people know they need to move, but they quit before they even start thanks to all the cultural shaming and daily downloads they're consuming. They think, *why bother?*

We get it. You're under constant cultural pressure to fit into some predetermined definition of beauty and fitness and health. You turn your gaze upon the health and wellness experts, and you see these men and women with lush locks, and buff bodies, and like 5 percent body fat. Even if it seems so far away from where you are, you still want to know their secrets.

We'll tell you their secret. We go to all the big health and wellness conferences. We know many people in the industry. We see behind the curtain, and guess what?

Many of the people you idolize are spiritually dead. Many of the people who lead seemingly perfect, healthy lives, are trapped in their own health crisis, just as exhausted and burned out as you.

We see these people without all the makeup and Botox, without the airbrushed, digitally altered photos that you see on Instagram. A lot of these people lead messy lives.

One of the biggest secrets to the health-celebrity world is the slathering on of testosterone—women and men alike. People use testosterone lotion. (Yeah, it's a thing.)

Is this everyone? No. There are some incredible people doing extraordinary work, offering killer insight and advice, and helping many people overcome their biggest challenges. These are the people showing up in this book and in our documentaries.

"Take what you need, and leave the rest," is apt advice, so if some tip or insight doesn't resonate, ring true, or work for you, it's okay to let it go. Except, many of us aren't taught this. We're not taught to tap into ourselves for the answers and to learn what our unique bodies need. Instead, we're taught to compare and contrast ourselves against unrealistic, unattainable images.

This narrative that you've been living can be one of the biggest energy drains, zapping your zest and vitality. We want to stop the madness. We want you to ditch the story you've been unconsciously living.

Energy Drain #2:
You've Got Too Much Storage and Not Enough Burn

Your body is designed to be an energy producing *and* burning machine.

For some people, they're not burning nearly enough energy, and that's leading them to feel exhausted. It can also lead to extra pounds. Some of the challenge here is cultural. We have so much start/stop time in America. We hurry to our cars so we can sit in traffic for an hour. We sprint up the stairs to work because we're late, only to sit at our desks without moving all day.

Maybe we spend an hour at the gym. We put on our acceptable gym clothing and move in acceptable gym ways like hitting the treadmill or doing some bicep curls. We get a little sweaty, count some calories on our devices, and that's it. We race home, only to eat dinner and lounge on the couch with our honeys while binging a show. Then we go to bed and rinse and repeat the next day.

This is what exercise and movement means in our modern world.

It's not that getting on a treadmill for an hour a day is bad. Kudos for getting to the gym when you have a million and one responsibilities and demands for your attention!

The problem is that that one hour is probably not enough.

We are animals that have evolved around constant movement on a three-dimensional plane. We were hunters and gatherers who climbed hills, scrambled over boulders, and waded through rippling streams in search of food and shelter. When we shifted to farming, we spent days plowing fields, harvesting vegetables, tending to sheep and cattle, building fences, chopping wood, and so much more.

We moved all the time, and when the sun set, we collapsed because we were actually exhausted and needed to rest our aching muscles.

But we've flipped that script. Our labor-saving devices have robbed us of our birthright—constant movement.

Hamsters get their wheels—humans have planet Earth as our playground. To get out of this exhaustion mess, you have to start moving, then you have to build steady movement into your day by hacking your environment. That's the formula for success.

Energy Drain #3:
You're Not Stressing Your Muscle Enough

There was a famous study done by researchers in Finland[2] that took identical twins and put them in different training programs. One trained for a marathon, the other in high-intensity interval training (HIIT)—that's sprinting, jumping, and building muscles. The researchers had to stop the experience because the health of the marathoner was crashing while the other twin was just getting bigger and buffer.

The takeaway: forget taking the same spinning class or lumbering for an hour on that grimy elliptical five times a week. Cardio-only training doesn't work. Sure, it's an important part of the exercise and movement mix, and you definitely want to get your heart rate up. But if you really want to become the lean, mean, energy-producing *and* burning machine you were born to be, you have got to focus on building lean muscle.

Muscle is the densest tissue of mitochondria. Remember, mito-chondria are your energy-producing machines, so if you want a big life and to have the energy to live it, build your muscles. This will give you the ability to produce more energy.

For your energy to keep pumping and you to feel healthy, your mitochondria have to be able to cope with the stressors of life and maintain what's called *homeostasis*. Basically, homeostasis is your ability to remain stable despite environmental changes—so, whether it's 40 or 80 degrees out, your body temperature should remain the same.

There are all kinds of things your mitochondria have to cope with to maintain homeostasis: weather, physical activity, and other stressors, including mental and emotional stress. Your mitochondria's ability to cope with all of this has everything to do with why Ari Whitten calls this the *mitochondrial reserve capacity*.[3] In short, their resilience threshold.

"The bigger and stronger your mitochondria, and the more of them you have, the higher your resilience to the stress of life," Ari explained. "But if your mitochondria have shrunken, shriveled, or become weak and fragile, the easier it is for stressors like poor nutrition, sleep deprivation, environmental toxins, and psycholog-ical stress to overwhelm the system and exceed the mitochondrial reserve capacity. That's when you start to get shutdown of the mito-chondria. You start to get fatigue. You start to get the emergence of lots of other symptoms."[4]

By building lean muscle, you're making your mitochondria bigger and stronger and better able to cope with whatever stressors come at you.

You also get another extraordinary benefit with lean muscle—*mitochondrial biogenesis*. "Your body can create more mitochondria from scratch," said Ari.[5] You aren't just getting bigger and stronger mitochondria; now you're getting more of those suckers too.

To get the lean muscle mass you need, you have to put your body under some stress.

We know that sounds counter to what is often said. Stress is supposed to be a bad thing, and in many contexts, it is. Quick history lesson: the word we use for *stress* was coined by a guy named Hans Selye in the 1950s, and he had two variations. This *stress* we immediately think about, which is all the shit flying at us, and *eustress* (prounounced *YOU-stress*), now also known as *hormetic stress*, which is a positive stress response.

Strength training is a really obvious example. If you're lifting the right way—something that's heavy but not too heavy—you're actually damaging your muscles. (Bear with us. We promise, this is a good thing.) The weight isn't enough to cause injury, but it's a relatively low and manageable form of damage. It might show up as sore muscles the next day.

Now when your body goes to heal that minor damage, it comes in and builds some new stronger muscle fibers, along with repairing the existing ones. Remember "No pain, no gain"? Well, this is where it comes from.

Hormetic stressors used to be a very natural part of life for our ancestors. We're talking about the stressors of running and jumping and hunting and using their bodies to survive. But we've become accustomed to our creature comforts, our high-calorie foods, our temperature-controlled homes, and the ease of living. Our modern lifestyles have created environments where we don't stress ourselves physically.

We have to voluntarily introduce it, and exercise is one of the most potent ways. Exposing it to cold and hot temperatures, fasting, breathing exercises, and ingesting certain herbs can also create a beneficial, or hormetic, stress response.

For most people, exercise is the path of least resistance and the one they're already familiar with. The trick is introducing just the *right amount of stress*.

If you introduce too much, your body gets overwhelmed. If you introduce too little, your body is underwhelmed. What you want is to find the "whelm" line, the "if it doesn't kill you, it makes you stronger."

To be clear, we're talking muscles, not joints. If you're going "no pain, no gain" and your knee hurts . . . that's just an orthopedic visit. Your muscles will fatigue and fail—you want them to get a little sore and tired. Joints, though, aren't designed for that type of stress, so a sharp pain in your knee or shoulder isn't fatigue. It's injury.

But if you push yourself every day where your legs get stronger and stronger, then you'll have an epigenetic expression. An epigenetic expression might involve your genes recognizing that you are not someone who is sitting and chilling all the time, so they signal to your body, "Hey, this animal is doing it. It's not dying, it's growing, and this buck's going to own the mountain, so we better start building muscle *now*."

You're tearing muscle fiber when you hit this "whelm" line. As your body recovers, and the muscle grows, now you adapt into a bigger, smarter, stronger animal, with more energy to use.

Energy Drain #4: You've Forgotten How to Move

Many of us have no idea how to move our bodies. American culture has largely beaten it out of us. From a young age, we're taught to sit still, be quiet, don't fidget, and stop running, jumping, dancing, playing . . . you name it. And we're paying the price for it.

Movement is everything you as a human being, as part of the animal kingdom, were born to do. Movement is natural, but often it's not something that's celebrated, supported, or encouraged.

Today, many of us live in cultures that can make it very difficult to leave our wolf packs and push against the ingrained teachings, whether that's from our families, educational centers, society, or even major religious institutions that have stigmatized the lower centers of our bodies. You know, where the sex stuff goes on. From an early age, many of us are taught to cover up, tamp down, and not to move our bodies in a "provocative" way, let alone acknowledge they exist.

As a result, it's like we don't have the permission for our bodies to feel the way they need to feel or move the way they need to move, unless it's following the guidelines of "acceptance." For example, neither of us grew up learning how to move our hips or asses. Until we started studying and practicing in the health and wellness spaces, we moved like robots. We had no idea what was going on beneath our necks, and this is true for many people today.

If you don't use your full mobility, you lose it. And when that's gone, you lose pathways to restoring your energy. If you want to experience the vitality of life, you have to break free from these cultural learnings and remember what it's like to move in your body.

Relearning how to move can be life changing. Pedram once worked with a San Diego neurologist who treats kids suffering from learning and behavioral disorders.

She would ask these kids to get on the ground and show her how they creep around. Well, they couldn't do it. They had been moved to bouncers before they were allowed to be blobs of flesh on the floor who learned how to move. They had missed that pivotal developmental step and developed cognitive dysfunction—their brains didn't work right and their energy was messed up.

Here's where it gets really wild. The neurologist asked the mothers to get on the ground with their kids to help teach them how to creep. Mom gets on the floor with Baby, and as Baby starts getting better, suddenly Mom is like, "hey, my migraines have gone away," and "hey, my shoulder pain is gone."

Mom didn't need prescription drugs. She didn't need surgery. She just needed to remember how to naturally move her body.

This isn't just for people who aren't moving. It's just as important for physically active folks too. If you're someone who does the same workout day in and day out, then you're likely one twist away from throwing something out.

Energy Drain #5: You Think Exercise Is a Destination

Some people work out because they're ashamed of their bodies. They're ashamed of how they look, how they feel, and what other people will say. It doesn't even matter what the number on the scale reads. You can be overweight, playing with 10 pounds, maintaining, or wanting to put weight on—it's all a shame game.

We set goals like getting ripped in three to four months, or losing 20 pounds in two. Then we tear it up, working out six days a week, committing wholeheartedly to achieving the goal, and sometimes we do. We build that muscle, we lose that weight, and we feel like we've conquered the mountain. But what comes after we meet our goals? Unless we set another, it's easy to fall back into old unhealthy patterns, which is what, unfortunately, happens to many of us. We realize our workouts have become exhausting—the pace and intensity are unsustainable.

For many of us, we see exercise as a chore, just one more thing to knock off our to-do list for the day. We get in and get out as quickly as possible because we don't want to be at gym, on the bike path, at the Zumba class, lifting weights, or jogging on our treadmill at home.

The problem isn't the exercising and movement; it's your attitude. It's how you see exercise and movement as a part of your life. The people who have the healthiest relationship with exercising and movement do it because they *love it*. It's something they look forward to (most of the time). It's enjoyable. It's fun, and they feel great during and after their workouts.

They see working out, exercising, and moving their bodies as a journey, not a destination.

When you see it as a journey and something that you can enjoy, then the thought of working out doesn't seem exhausting or boring. It seems like an adventure that you can direct and change at any time.

Energy Drain #6:
You're Overtraining and Getting Injured

Earlier we explained how exercising is one of the best intentional stressors you can place on your body. You're asking your body to meet a goal, to rev your heart rate, and get stronger.

Here's the catch: when you put that stress on your body, you better have enough energy in the tank to get you through. Otherwise, you're stressing the system too much, and this can lead to exhaustion.

We've seen people cranking on the CrossFit classes day after day, wondering why they're so exhausted. Part of the answer is they're running on empty. The other part is that they're not allowing their bodies to actually heal and recover, and build the muscle density they need.

To build lean muscle mass and get all the awesome benefits of strengthening and multiplying your mitochondria, your body needs some inflammation. We know, in the last chapter we talked about what a number inflammation does on your body. But with healthy exercise, it's a good thing.

It only stays good, though, if you allow the inflammation to subside. That's when you let the muscle fibers that have torn heal and knit back stronger than before. But when you're pounding out the workouts six days a week, the inflammation builds and builds.

When you're constantly inflamed, you're at a greater risk for injury and exhaustion. "If inflammation is not allowed to subside, if that CrossFitter finishes their workout and comes back the next morning and the next and the next for six days, that's an example where inflammation builds," explained Ben Greenfield, fitness author and personal trainer to pro athletes from UFC to the NHL, NBA, and NFL. "That's where collagen and elastin break down and scar tissue forms around a joint like an ankle, which becomes immobile and a pain point. That's a situation where the body actually becomes exhausted in its attempts to repair the inflammation that's occurring day after day. By exhaustion, I mean a loss of creatine, a loss of ATP, a depletion of glucose, a depletion of fatty acids, a depletion of endogenous built-in antioxidants responsible for quelling that chronic inflammation."[6]

Sometimes the overtraining comes from trying to do too much too soon, and your body can't handle it. We live in a culture where a lot of us don't want to work hard for a living; we just want to be instant millionaires. Or, we wake up one morning and for some reason—maybe a big life event or someone fat shamed us—we decide today is the day we're finally going to do something about our fitness.

We go to a boot camp class or we run three miles and we pull our hamstrings. Then we're down for six months, and we've gained 50 pounds.

Recognizing the need to move more and bring fitness back into your lifestyle is incredible, and everyone should be applauded for that. And there is wisdom in going slowly, in building up, and meeting yourself where you're at, especially if movement has not been a regular part of your life. There is no such thing as a shortcut to getting six-pack abs, bulging biceps, or a tight butt.

Personal Quest (Nick)

About a year ago, I was experiencing some pretty severe lower back pain. My second child, Rowan, was about a year and a half old, so I spent a lot of time carrying him around on my hip. And you know how these things go: the pain grows and you don't even notice it. Until I realized I had, like, five jars of Tiger Balm around the house and most of them were half-empty. This wasn't good.

But one night I was in charge of watching the kids, because my wife, Michelle, was out for the evening. We were having a dance party, and a salsa song came on. The boys were doing their thing, and I started moving my hips, getting into it. I was just in my zone, but I noticed that when I started doing some hip and butt stuff (the things you have to do in order to be a remotely convincing salsa dancer), I was able to stretch a part of my lower back that I'd never reached before, not even with yoga. With salsa, your butt starts leading your body, instead of your brain, and you engage parts of your body that don't always get used. These exaggerated movements were helping my pelvis unlock itself.

So, hell yes, I played more Latin tracks, and my pain was gone within 10–20 minutes.

Full disclosure: we dance our faces off in the Polizzi household. It's useful, and it's fun.

TESTS

The same tests that we suggested in Chapters 2 and 3 that you get from your functional medicine practitioner apply here as well. Exercise needs energy. Energy needs mitochondrial function. Mitochondria need nutrients and a balanced microbiome. Some of the nutrient levels your doctor may test for include:

Plasma Amino Acids

Looking at your amino acid levels is essential for building lean muscle mass. You can't build new tissue if you are missing one of the amino acid building blocks. Make sure you have your practitioner track your branched chain amino acid/BCAA levels (leucine, isoleucine, and valine), along with your glutamic acid, glutamine, tryptophan, and arginine. If any of these are deficient, you will be fighting a major uphill battle when exercising.

Mineral Testing for Magnesium

Magnesium is the king for energy and therefore essential for exercise. Looking at red blood cell/RBC magnesium will give you a clue on your magnesium status but is not 100 percent accurate in determining your current need for magnesium. Taking a supplement or eating lots of magnesium-rich foods like green leafy veggies, nuts, seeds, and beans may be important while exercising. If you are sweating during your exercise routines, be sure to add in lots of potassium-rich foods like avocados, kiwi, coconut water, beans, and sweet potatoes.

B Vitamins

When you are tearing down muscle tissues and building newer and stronger tissues, you will be using some enzymes that need B vitamins to do the job right. One B vitamin, vitamin B_6, becomes really important at this time. Your practitioner can track the kynurenate and xanthurenate levels on your organic acids panel to see where your current status is and whether supplementation might be necessary.

(The amino acid, mineral, and organic acid tests are all included when your practitioner orders an ION or NutrEval Plasma test from Genova Diagnostics.)

THE ENERGY REMEDIES

Energy Remedy #1: Embrace a New Narrative

You have been brainwashed into thinking that the number on the scale, your jean size or muscle size, how you look, or what other people tell you about your looks are the all-important metrics. They're not. Those are external. You are so much more. We want you to take all the societal and cultural bullshit and let it go.

Fuck how you look.

What matters is what's happening *inside* your body. What matters is how you're *feeling*. What you need to care about is burning fat, powering your cells, having a ton of energy, and feeling amazing. The most compelling, attractive, and interesting people are those who move through life with such energy and vibrancy and grace that you can't help but feel alive in their presence.

Exercise and movement are about helping you to achieve inward transformations. It's about helping you from the inside out, so you radiate energy, and live the good life—one that's long, happy, and healthy.

Embracing a new narrative and unhooking from the dastardly stories you've been told may not come easy. Deprogramming may take some effort, time, and practice. But it's so worth it. When you let go of all the bullshit you've been buying into, you will experience true freedom and connection with the true MVP—you. When you get to the point when you feel great in your body, when you've become a fat-burning machine, and your energy levels are humming, the side effects can be fat loss, beautiful butts and abs, and a healthy glowing skin.

Focus on how you move through the world and on learning how to move with the undertones of the universe. When you do this, you reject the cultural, energy-stealing narrative, and instead tap into infinite energy of the cosmos.

Energy Remedy #2 and #3: Build Lean Muscle

If you want to become a lean, mean energy-producing and energy-burning machine, then you've got to get your *basal metabolic rate* (BMR) up. We're talking burning calories while you rest, like while you sleep, watch TV, or sit at your desk.

The good news is you can figure out your BMR yourself. The Harris-Benedict equation can help estimate your basal metabolic rate. It uses variables like height, weight, age, and gender, and is more accurate than estimating your calorie needs based on body weight alone. Here's how it works:

Women: BMR = 655 + (4.35 x weight in pounds) + (4.7 x height in inches) - (4.7 x age in years)

Men: BMR = 66 + (6.23 x weight in pounds) + (12.7 x height in inches) - (6.8 x age in years)

To raise your BMR, focus on boosting your *active metabolic rate*. These are calories you burn due to physical activity—so jogging, yoga, hiking, etc. You know, when you're active.

The cool thing is that when your active metabolic rate is nice and high, your resting metabolic rate is higher too. So even when you're chilling, your body burns more calories.

When you get these rates up, you're turning on the engine and signaling to your body, "Hey, this animal is alive and using calories, so that lunch she just ate? Burn it off as energy. Don't you dare store it as fat."

By building *lean muscle mass*, you raise your BMR. Lean muscle is where your mitochondria are most concentrated, and you need plenty of hard-working mitochondria to keep your metabolism at an optimal level. "The more muscle mass you have, the more capacity you have to generate energy," said Dr. Stephanie Estima. "From an energetic and a metabolism standpoint, the more muscle you have, the more efficient you are at disposing of glucose."[7]

Right now, odds are you're toast. Your mitochondria are likely weak, so you have to start slowly, stacking incrementally and building your muscles. We don't expect that you're going to dive into a massive training regimen today. But you deserve to know what you're working toward and what kind of balanced exercise and movement that you want to one day experience.

We don't want you to be a mindless zombie who kills it on the elliptical or treadmill, going at a slow-steady pace. There is a place for endurance and building stamina, but if you do the same cardio routine day after day, you won't push your muscles to the "whelm" line we mentioned earlier. Don't ditch cardio entirely, but use it wisely as part of a balanced workout regimen.

Life is about balance. Seek it with your exercise too. Each week, aim for a mix of:

1. **Cardio.** This is a steady pace for a longer duration of time or distance to build endurance, or the short sprints that get your heart rate pumping.

2. **Strength Training.** This is lifting heavier weights at lower repetitions.

3. **Resistance Training.** This is where you're building muscle by using your body weight or you're lifting lighter weights for more repetitions.

4. **Rest and Recovery.** You support your body healing from inflammation when you give yourself a day or two of rest or gentle recovery exercises, which can include yoga, walking, swimming, tai chi, or qigong.

Mix and match your week with the stuff you enjoy. If you like jogging, then jog one day for distance, do some strength training the next, add a yoga or tai chi or qigong class, and then throw in a High Intensity Interval Training (HIIT) session or two.

HIIT workouts have become very popular in recent years and can be a great way to build muscle. It's cardio and fat-burning rolled into one epic exercise. It's perfect for someone who has only 20 minutes to work out. With HIIT workouts, you go hard for 15 or 30 seconds, then you rest for 3 minutes. Repeat that three times, and you have just activated your primal exercise system.

You can do HIIT on a treadmill, elliptical, rowing machine, bike, or outdoors at a high school track or park. For example, pretend you're a deer and sprint as if a jaguar's chasing you for 30 seconds. Stop, pant, shake it out, and release all the adrenaline for three minutes, then sprint again for 30 seconds, rest for three minutes, and rinse and repeat two more times. Then go home. If 30 seconds is too long, no problem, start with 10 or 15 seconds, and if you need to rest for five minutes, do it! If doing three cycles is too much, start with one or two rounds, then gradually, as the weeks go by, you can increase the length of your sprint or the number of rounds, and/or decrease the time between resting and sprinting.

And if sprinting is too much, walk at a brisk pace or pedal just a bit faster. All you're aiming for is to vary the speed to get that heart rate up and your muscles working.

Remember, there is no race. There is no "right" way to do this. We know that sometimes when you're starting out, you can feel disappointed and you may beat up on yourself for "not being faster or stronger" or able to "go as long." We've all been there, no matter our energy or fitness levels. All that matters is you're out there, moving your body, doing whatever you can do, and taking it one day at a time. Slow and steady progress will make a huge difference in your energy levels.

Last point on HIIT workouts: they aren't meant to be done every day—twice, maybe three times per week, max.

Once it all starts feeling "easy" (we know, exercise is never really easy, but when your body feels like it's not being challenged, then it's time to step up the intensity), do more reps, go a minute or two longer, increase the incline or speed, add a little more weight, or change up the workout. You're aiming for sore muscles.

Shoot for the "whelm" and you'll be good.

Energy Remedy #4: Relearn How to Move

All of us can benefit from reconnecting to our most primal instincts and movements. It may sound silly, but just getting on the floor and crawling around could make a difference—just be sure to tell your sweetie what's up so they don't look at you like you've lost your mind.

Or you could start by just paying attention to the ordinary ways you move every day. Next time you're out doing some yard work or hammering away at a home project, pay attention to your body's mechanics. We all know "lift with your legs, not your back," but what does that mean? Are you engaging your core? Are you keeping your spine aligned? Are you using your muscles or your joints to do the work?

Some folks who are really stiff may want to visit a physical therapist. It can make a world of difference. Physical therapists can teach you movements and stretches, and help you create programs to strengthen and improve flexibility based on where your body is right now.

Alternatively, the Feldenkrais Method is a blockbuster program that's designed to help you remember how to move your body by taking you back to some of the first movements you ever did on this planet.

But you don't need to get super science-y. Don't be shy checking out exercise classes that promote gentle movement, stretching, and flexibility. Yoga and Pilates could be great starters for you. If you've never done either, check out beginner classes in your area. (Note: We said beginner. Don't dive right into an intermediate or advanced class. Give your body a chance to learn.)

And take a dance class! Guys, we're talking to you too. If you think dancing is the dude-at-a-concert head nod, or a gentle kind of bopping sway, there's *a lot* more to it. Dancing is a great workout, but more importantly it asks you to move your body in ways that are outside the boxes we often place ourselves in. Swing dancing, salsa, hip-hop—whatever you're into, get into it! (And we can tell you, your sweetie will thank you.)

Energy Remedy #5: Go for the Love of It

When you look at exercising as a lifestyle and journey instead of as a way to achieve just a goal, everything changes. Take the Tarahumara tribe, an indigenous people living in Chihuahua, Mexico. They live to run, and they run to live. They're known for running 200-mile ultra-marathons. To them, running is a part of reverence and appreciation for life. When they're running, it might as well be the rest of their life.

It's as though they run for the love of running, for the joy of it. It's their way of connecting themselves with the earth, with the harmony of life, and with the life force stored within. They get energy from these experiences.

They're not the only ones. Watch kids. They're constant balls of motion, most likely burning tons of calories without even thinking about it or trying to. They're just having fun. We need to remind ourselves to have fun too. Movement can be fun, and your fun can be movement.

Life is hard enough. Why make movement and exercise hard too? Instead, make this easy. If all you have is 45 minutes to work out, choose something you *want* to do and is fun for you, not something a fitness magazine says you should. Nick can run seven or eight miles and feel good while he's doing it, but he doesn't enjoy it, and it takes him two days to recover. Instead, he loves lifting weights in the gym or doing high-intensity workouts. Pedram loves playing basketball, going for hikes, and practicing qigong. For you, maybe yoga is your thing, or swimming, or judo, or biking, or dancing, or rock climbing, or hiking, or dodgeball, or running. The list of activities and ways to move is endless.

Maybe you don't know what exercises and movement you love. That's okay. It means you get to discover it. You don't need to have a structured workout either—you just need to move, build lean muscle, and bring more joy into your life. You could throw a spontaneous dance party in the kitchen, play tag with your kids, or go for a walk after dinner.

When you start feeling some joy and fun again, you'll feel lighter, and you'll feel the universe moving through you. You'll feel like you have energy again—because you do.

You don't have to go it alone, either. Exercising with a pal can up the enjoyment quota, as well as keep you accountable. No matter what you may think or worry about or have been told, you're never too old or out of shape to fall in love with exercise. You may have to pace yourself, start slowly, and regain some strength, stamina, flexibility, endurance, but remember, this is a journey—you have time.

Energy Remedy #6: Meet Yourself Where You're At

Let's be straight. You're exhausted, so you have no business doing an aggressive exercise regimen right now. Every time you fail a New Year's resolution or bail on a workout, it seems like you prove to yourself that you can't keep your word and you're a failure.

So, first order of business: *cut that shit out.*

You don't have the mitochondrial capacity to do that level of intensity. You may not even feel like working out and moving your body. And your mind's awful self-talk creates the negative circuitry that reinforces the lack of movement, which reinforces less energy and motivation. You have to start somewhere, and that somewhere is meeting yourself where you're at.

There is no shame in this. Honestly, it takes mad courage and bravery to be this person.

When patients came into Pedram's clinic with deep exhaustion, the remedy was simple: walking. Seriously. That's all he had people do at first—a 15-minute walk per day, that's it, for a week, then they talked.

If his patient came back and was like, "Hey man, that wiped me out," then he had them cut it down to five minutes a day and a little bit of stretching.

Starting where you're at could be doing 5 minutes of qigong and a 10-minute walk every day for 100 days. If that's all you've got in the tank, that's fine. You'll live to fight another day, and you will grow stronger. After 100 days, you'll build to maybe a 10-minute qigong practice and a 20-minute walk and some wall squats.

Incremental progress wins the game, but start at the right level *for you*, even if that's by taking two more steps today than you did yesterday. You want to exercise so that you feel slightly tired and like you've exerted yourself—but you feel revitalized within 20–30 minutes. If you're still feeling tapped out an hour later, then you've done too much.

And then, add 10 percent more to your routine every week. Again, if it feels like too much, scale it back. Listen to your body.

This approach builds confidence. Doing the small things and doing them predictably and in a disciplined way is a huge part of creating a healthy mindset and relationship with exercise, movement, and your body.

Keep in mind, just because you say you're going to work out for 45 minutes, doesn't mean you have to. If you don't have the gas in the tank and your body's screaming at you to stop, listen. If after two exercises, you're beat, let it go.

The same holds true on the flipside. If you get into a workout and you're crushing it and your body feels great, go longer.

Your body knows what it needs. Tune in. Listen. Learn its subtle signals and we guarantee you'll feel a helluva lot better, happier, and filled with vitality. This is a lifestyle. You want exercise and movement to be a part of your daily life, just like drinking water.

SOLUTION

All right, so Amy had a rough time at Power Yoga. Guess what? Yoga's not for everyone.

Amy didn't find her solution right away, and when she did find it, she didn't even realize she had. She just one day noticed that she was feeling better, and then eventually she noticed that she was happier with her body.

How did it happen?

Amy's dog was overweight, and the vet told her he needed longer walks. She figured they both could use the extra steps, so she added an extra thirty minutes to their strolls. At first it was hard—both she and her dog were panting at the end and just wanted to lie down and sleep. She kept going, and before long she found that they had more energy at the end of their walk, not less. They even started running a little together, just for the joy of it.

She also started going on more hikes with her granddaughter. It was a ritual they both really enjoyed, but after a while they got bored with the same old one-mile loop. They got adventurous and hiked for two miles, then four. Then they did it every other week, instead of just once a month.

The ladies from book group noticed the change, not just in how she looked, but in Amy's energy—in who she was. She laughed more, and she was eager to go out and do things. And one day, just for the hell of it, she went back to that yoga class with Mary Ann. It was still long and tiring, but this time she rested when she needed to and modified when her body wasn't ready for something. And at the end of the class, she felt great.

PERSONAL CHALLENGE

Try something that you've always wanted to this week. Martial arts? Yoga? Rock climbing? Dance? Surfing? Cross-country skiing? Biking? Anything goes. Just be mindful about your skill and fitness level. Go slowly and pace yourself. If you need to sign up for a beginner or introductory class or work with an instructor, do it. Your goal is to connect joy and fun with movement, and you get to decide what that looks like.

CHAPTER 5

Sleep and Recovery

Brian could pinpoint exactly when his sleep troubles began. He just had no idea how to fix it.

It all started when he took on a new position at his company. He was in his early forties and had accepted a job that paid more, but that came with more people to manage and more responsibilities.

From the start, Brian felt like there was never enough time for him to get everything done during the day. After he and his wife put the kids to bed at 7:30 P.M., he would open his laptop and work until at least 10, sometimes 10:30.

By the time he called it a day, he wasn't tired. He needed to unwind and relax. His wife would usually go to bed before him, and hoping to just be near her, he'd crawl into bed and turn on the television, keeping the volume low so she could sleep.

Around midnight, he'd shut off the television. But he'd lie awake, staring at the ceiling. His body felt tired, but he couldn't sleep. His mind raced with thoughts about what had happened that day and what was coming tomorrow.

Sometimes, as he lay there, he'd remember an email that needed a response, so he'd roll over, grab his phone from the nightstand, and quickly fire off his answer. If it was slightly more complicated, he'd get back to his desk and go way later.

Most nights, he didn't fall asleep until 1 or 2 A.M. When his alarm buzzed at 5:30 A.M., it was hard to get out of bed. The days began to get even tougher for him—but that's what coffee was for. He'd drink it morning, noon, and sometimes after dinner just to keep him going.

Brian had promised his wife this was only temporary. He just needed to ease into the job, and once he felt more comfortable, he'd take his foot off the gas.

That was five years ago.

Brian's been working with a business coach to better manage his time, and he's put up some work boundaries, but his sleep is wrecked. He can't fall asleep before midnight, and when he does, he just tosses and turns.

He knows this isn't healthy for him—he just doesn't know how to turn around this sinking ship.

THE PROBLEM

"Sleep is under-recognized as playing such an important role in our energy," said Dr. David Perlmutter.[1]

Sleep puts energy in the bank. Too bad most of us are broke. When we sleep, we recover the energy we burned that day. If we're not sleeping, then we're not recovering.

Like exercise, we know we need it, but something is stopping us from getting the sleep we desperately need. We're not talking about very valid reasons that can keep us up like our kid wakes us up at 1 A.M. with the stomach flu or a bad dream—we've both been there, done that.

We're talking about the string of sleepless nights, of lying awake tossing and turning, of being unable to fall asleep or stay asleep. That's what's destroying our sleep and needs fixing. Sleep is so critical to your energy levels that it's actually one of the first, if not the first, areas a functional medicine doctor will examine in their patients.

For most people, it's not like they don't want to sleep; it's that they can't. And if they do sleep, it's not *restful sleep*. In this chapter, we want to help you better understand *why* good sleep may be eluding you. At the end of this chapter, we're going to give you some possible remedies to help turn around your slumber challenges.

We wrote "possible" because solving these issues can get complicated. Like so much in this book, your path to fixing sleep is uniquely yours.

There is no formula that works for everyone, and nowhere is this lesson clearer than in this chapter. Sometimes just making small changes to the bedroom like adding blackout curtains and keeping the room cooler is enough to help. Sometimes meditating, journaling, or reading an hour before bed is all it takes. And sometimes just falling asleep an hour earlier and stacking a few nights like that in a row makes the difference.

But if you're already on the breadline of sleep, if you haven't had a good night's rest in months or years, then drinking kava tea, deep breathing, or shutting off all devices an hour before bedtime probably won't cut it. They're part of your solution, but you'll need to take a "multi-system" approach for tougher cases.

"Sometimes you fix sleep issues by making sure you get someone's brain healthier," said Dr. Datis Kharrazian. "Sometimes you fix sleep issues by making sure that they get enough glucose throughout the day so they have enough glycogen, so they can get through the night and not have a hypoglycemic event and wake up. Sometimes you fix sleep issues by having them change their lifestyle so their stress levels go down, so they can finally fall asleep. Sometimes they have to exercise, to burn off stress, so they can actually fall asleep. Fixing sleep issues can be a host of things, not just one thing."[2]

This could be you. If it is, you can and should still try the remedies in this chapter. You never know if one or two holds the key for you.

If you try every remedy, and they're duds, don't despair. You may have to work on your gut first, or address nutrient deficiencies, or look at your hormones and adrenals. This may mean you have to find a functional medical practitioner or someone who can help walk this journey with you. That's okay. These doctors exist. Use the information in this chapter to feel confident and comfortable talking with them, so you can make informed decisions about your health.

The answers you seek are here. Don't let anyone tell you that you're fated for a lifetime of poor sleeping, because you aren't.

Stay hopeful. Stay alert. Stay committed to your energy recovery, and trust that you can and will find the right path to better sleep.

THE ENERGY DRAINS

Energy Drain #1: You Never Reach REM or Deep Sleep

More than a third of American adults are not getting enough sleep on a regular basis.[3] We know a lot of people who say their bodies are unique and they only need five or six hours of sleep. And for some people that's true—but most of the time, it's bullshit. For the vast majority of people, our bodies need at least seven hours.[4] Eight hours is even better.

But it's not just the number of hours; it's the quality too.

There are four stages of sleep with REM falling in between, and you'll cycle through these stages over and over. You start off going through them in sequence, but after you've made it to Stage 4, you usually cycle back and forth between 3 and 2, with REM coming in now and again.

Stage 1

This is when you're in bed, you're tired, and you've just shut off the light. Your mind has started to release its conscious hold, and you'll have a period of dreaminess—much like daydreaming, but with a little less control. This is called the *Alpha state*. Alpha brain waves are sort of the "frequency bridge" between our conscious mind and the unconscious mind. People who practice meditation tend to spend a lot of time here in this restful place.

It's easy to get startled out of it. You know how sometimes when you feel like you're just about to fall asleep, you experience a sudden physical jolt or a feeling of falling? This is called a *hypnogogic hallucination*, and it's totally normal—it's just part of falling asleep sometimes.

Stage 2

After Alpha, you begin to enter Theta sleep. This is still really light, and somewhere between being awake and asleep. Theta brain wave is, in a way, the border between being conscious and unconscious.

Stage 1 and 2 together usually last for about 5 to 10 minutes total.

Stage 3
Now your body begins to shut down. Your brain produces a period of rapid, rhythmic brain wave activity called *Sleep Spindles*. Your body temperature drops, and your heart rate slows down.

This stage lasts around 20 minutes.

Stage 4
Stage 4 is Delta sleep—it's deep sleep that lasts for about 30 minutes. This is when your brain is really resting, with some long, slow brain waves.

REM
REM sleep comes and goes throughout, interrupting the various stages. Dreaming occurs here, as it is a fairly active state of sleep. REM stands for rapid eye movement, but that's not all that moves—your respiration rate increases, as does your brain activity. REM sleep is also a form of paralysis. Although your brain is going on all sorts of adventures, your body is definitely not along for the ride. During REM sleep, your voluntary muscles in your arms and legs cannot move (though your involuntary muscles like your heart and gut can carry on just fine). You know how sometimes you're trying to run away in a dream, but you just can't? Well, it's because you literally can't.

Each of these stages is absolutely critical to your energy levels. Without Stages 1 and 2, you can't make it to Stages 3 and 4. If you don't make it to Stages 3 and 4, you're clinically screwed—you're not getting enough REM, and you're not getting deep sleep.

Now let's look at what's going on during Stage 4.

According to the National Sleep Foundation, deep sleep supports memory consolidation—this is when short-term memory converts into long-term memory, and when long-term memory gets organized into "islands of memory" that are easier to access. Deep sleep also supports overall learning, and it's when the pituitary gland secretes hormones like the human growth hormone. (This is why it's so important that we make sure our kids get enough sleep. If we don't, they will be stunted, both body and mind.)

At the same time, your body is spending the energy it usually puts toward keeping the brain happy on things like repairing your immune and digestive systems, as well as any damaged tissues and muscles. Autophagy, or cell regeneration, energy restoration, and immune system support all take place during deep sleep.

The immune system is a big deal here. If you don't get enough sleep, your body can't make enough *cytokines*, a type of chemical compound that communicates from one immune cell to another. Cytokines are produced and released during sleep, and if you don't have them, you're effectively creating an immune response within your body. Not great.

Then what's going on during REM?

Well, first of all, you're working shit out. Our dreams are literally our way of processing our lives. Sometimes they can be really obvious, like when you have a classic stress dream about trying to get somewhere and always being prevented, or taking a test you didn't study for.

Other times your dreams are just weird, and who the hell knows what's going on in there. The subconscious is a mysterious place—but we all have to go there and play in all its wacky glory. A lack of dreaming, or even just poor dreaming, is strongly linked to emotional disturbance and to anxiety, depression, and other forms of mental illness,[5] most of which make it more difficult for you to sleep. Sleep begets sleep.

Aside from taking you on a psychedelic thrill ride of dreams, your brain is hard at work—it's cleaning itself like a car wash. During sleep, your brain shrinks by as much as 20 percent.[6] This is a good thing. It's getting rid of all the crud, all the stuff you don't need. Your lymphatic system sends fluid to the brain, washing away and draining all the gunk and buildup down your neck and to your liver to be detoxed. "We need eight hours of restorative sleep," advised Dr. David Perlmutter. "This is an incredibly important time for you to clean up your brain, and hit the reset button, so that the next day you can be energetic and more productive."[7]

When, and only when, you are in the deep Delta stage of sleep, you get this brainwash.

Without hitting REM and deep sleep, you're also at risk for weight gain. Research has also found a link between sleep and obesity.[8] Lack of sleep messes with the hormone *ghrelin*, which tells you when you're full. So not only do you wake up tired and without the cleaning your body and brain needed, you're also ravenous.

And lack of sleep may cause you to crave sugary, salty, or fatty foods that send you on a blood sugar rollercoaster, leading to weight gain and messing with your energy production. According to the Sleep Foundation, lack of sleep raises the levels of a lipid known as *endocannabinoid*. Does a word in there look familiar? It's because this lipid acts on the brain in much the same way marijuana/cannabis does, increasing your need for snacks, particularly cookies, candy, and chips. People who don't get enough sleep eat twice as much fat and more than 300 extra calories the next day than someone who got their eight hours the night before.

When we said you were clinically screwed if you're not sleeping, we meant it. And there's no way your energy levels will ever be where you want them to be without adequate sleep.

Energy Drain #2: You've Lost Your Circadian Rhythm

Sleep and energy are two sides of the same coin. They're linked by the *circadian rhythm*, which is like a 24-hour clock in your brain regulating hormones that affect your mood, energy levels, and the sleep-wake cycle.

And what keeps this clock running? Light.

For millions of years, our ancestors were guided only by the light of the sun and a little from the moon. The light went through their eyes, into their brains, and to their pineal glands. The pineal gland is charged with producing and regulating the hormone *melatonin*. Melatonin lets us know that it's time to go to sleep. It is also one of the most important antioxidants in the brain.

So, during the day, when the sun shines the brightest, it gives off a *blue light wavelength*. This blue light signals to our pineal gland,

"Hey, this animal needs to be awake, alert, active, and energetic as it forages and hunts. Get food now and rest when it can't gather."

When the sun sets, the light changes. It gives off *red light wavelengths*. Travel to Africa and you can really see how the light shifts color. There's a particular dust in the air, and the sun is this incredible red.

This red light stimulates the *serotonergic receptors of the prefrontal cortex*. This is the part of the brain that separates us from the chimps and has gifted us the capacities of higher moral reasoning, the negation of impulses, and better logic. Serotonin is the precursor to melatonin. It tells your pineal gland, "Hey, it's time for this animal to conserve energy and to fix the day's damage, so let's put them to bed." Cue melatonin.

Your melatonin should peak at night and in the early hours when you're asleep, and fall when you're exposed to morning light and during the daytime when you're working and active. This red-shifted light was critical to the development of our species. There's a theory that red-shifted light helped influence the evolution of our brains beyond monkeys.

Cliff's Notes version: blue light degrades melatonin and allows for an increase in cortisol and serotonin that keeps you awake and happy. Red light stimulates melatonin so you can fall asleep and stay asleep.

Century after century, our sleep-wake cycles were ruled by the sun rising and falling. Then electricity came, and everything changed. The modern world is almost perfectly designed to disrupt our circadian rhythms.

Our bodies are designed for lots of sunlight and staring at bright blue skies during the day. Instead, we've shifted to spending our days mostly indoors under dim and artificial light. And when the sun goes down and we shouldn't be exposed to any blue-shifted light, we're binging on it. Any blue light after sunset is harmful. But now we have computer screens, cell phones, TVs, tablets, and more that all emit blue light. The natural rhythms and swings that signal to our body to slow down and go to sleep are getting lost.

We've created a world where our bodies can no longer translate between light and dark, where they have no idea when they should be awake or asleep. And do we step outside to expose ourselves to natural sunlight within 30 minutes of waking? Most people don't, but they should. Letting the sun's rays hit your body is essential to normalizing and resetting the cycle of melatonin production.

We're also starting to learn more about electromagnetic frequencies (EMFs). Science is just beginning to understand how our gadgets and devices give off these frequencies that in some people affect their pineal glands and ability to produce melatonin.

Energy Drain #3: Your Nervous System Is in Fifth Gear

In the Kabbalah, all God's creations are equal except man was given stewardship of fire. Fire has tremendous responsibility.

Not only did our ancestors use fire to cook their food, it kept them safe and warm. When the sun set and the night rose, they would sit around the campfire and make music. Fire would keep away the predators, and it would keep these bands of humans together. They told stories and sang songs, developing rich cultures that we now take for granted.

On a primal level, fire kept us calm and relaxed. It gave us a bridge from our busy, work-filled days to when we entered the land of dreams. It helped us unwind from the day's struggles, giving off its own red light that soothed our nervous system and helped us move from our fight-or-flight state into rest and digest.

Today, there is no unwinding. There is no slowing down. There is only go, then go faster. There is only do, and do more.

So, when darkness comes calling, we can't quit. We feel lazy if we're sleeping. We have too much to figure out and so much work to do. We have bills to pay, emails from our boss to answer, and project deadlines to meet.

We have too much going on to give ourselves the luxury of rest, but that "luxury" is actually the key to getting more done. Rest could be the cheat codes to solving everything.

We understand the seductive pull of productivity. We're all for making the most of the time we're given on this here planet, but let's be realistic. If you're going to bed feeling like you didn't get enough done that day, then you're either hanging out at the watercooler too much *or* Dad's still looking over your shoulder psychologically, and you're trying to do too much.

Either way, it sucks your energy, because when you finally lie that weary head of yours down on the pillow, you can't slow your thoughts. You're worrying and agonizing over what happened during the day and what's coming at you tomorrow.

We call this being *wired and tired.*

Your body is exhausted and needs rest, but you can't slow your thoughts or your nervous system down enough to shift from the sympathetic, fight-or-flight state into the parasympathetic, rest-and-digest state.

If you're stressed out all day, cracked out on some coffee, and you're working on your laptop until midnight, do you honestly expect you can fall asleep in five minutes? That's like driving a car at 90 mph, slamming on the e-brake, and expecting everything's going to be fine.

If fight or flight is your modus operandi, and you're not giving yourself time to relax and get into a parasympathetic state, then you're screwed. You won't sleep and you will be exhausted.

A lot of people have to train their minds and nervous systems to slow down, to downshift into relax, digest, and heal. This means shutting off all your devices and eliminating bright lights one to two hours before you go to sleep. It means creating a quiet, meditative practice that helps your nervous system quiet itself, to come down from the fight-or-flight state, and learn what relaxation feels like.

Energy Drain #4: You Don't Have Enough Blood Sugar

If you have trouble staying asleep and you are waking up in the middle of the night with your heart racing, it can mean your adrenals are shot.

At night, your brain is going, "Okay, I'm going to do my detox, so everyone else, slow down. But I'm going to need some sugar (glucose) to burn, energy to do my repair work." Even though you're resting, your brain is hard at work, and it actually increases its need for glucose during deep sleep. And, for most people, general metabolism actually drops 10 to 15 percent during the night, sometimes going as low as 35 percent during stage 4 sleep.[9]

Ordinarily, this isn't a problem. Your glycogen reserves in your liver are supposed to handle this. If you have healthy adrenals, then your body goes, "Hey, the brain needs some more sugar; don't wake this gorilla up. Go get some sugar from the glycogen reserves." Your adrenals release a little cortisol, which signals to your liver to release the glycogen reserves, and all is well as you (gorilla) stay peacefully asleep.

But if you've overtaxed your adrenals by living in an eternal state of fight or flight (and, you know, by not getting enough sleep), then your adrenals aren't producing the necessary hormones at the rate you need them to. If you're at the point where there's just no cortisol to be had, then your body's going to wake you up.

Think of it like a bank. You have your checking account, a savings account, and your overdraft protection. Your brain's glucose is the checking account, and the adrenals are the savings account. If that savings account is empty, then you're going to get a phone call saying, "Sir, you have to put some glucose in here or your check's going to bounce."

No cortisol means your body's going to release some adrenaline. "Hey, gorilla, wake up. The brain is starving for sugar. Go get some food."

That's why you're waking up in the middle of the night with your heart racing.

Energy Drain #5: You're Making Poor Lifestyle Choices

For some people, poor sleep is caused simply by their evening choices and lifestyle habits. We've already touched on using devices, but there's more.

Here are some of the worst decisions we see people make. Study and learn them, so you won't make the same mistakes.

You're Drinking Too Much Coffee

When Pedram had a patient with insomnia, he told them they had to cut caffeine after 2 P.M. If their exhaustion was really bad, then they could have nothing after noon.

That's because caffeine stays in your system for a long time. If you're trying to unwind at 8 P.M. and you guzzled a mocha latte at 4

P.M., you'll have to wait until the caffeine has run its course before you can relax . . . and that can take a while. Caffeine has a half-life of 5–6 hours in most people, meaning it takes that long for just half the caffeine to leave your body—and in some people, it takes even longer.[10] So if you are wired and tired at night after drinking coffee even in the late morning, you may need to cut it out entirely.

That Adult Beverage Is Keeping You Up

It was a stressful day, and the kids are finally asleep. You have a little alone time with your sweetie, so what do you do? You unwind over a glass of wine or beer, or a bourbon nightcap. Maybe you just enjoyed one too many drinks at happy hour after work.

You go to bed with a slight buzz, thinking, *What's the big deal?*

It is a big deal because even a slight buzz can mess with your sleep. Alcohol can cause blood sugar spikes, which can make your heart race and your body sweat. You may have trouble staying asleep or sleeping soundly.

Your Bedroom Is a Concert Hall for Chaos

Sleeping and making love, that's all your bedroom should be for. It should be your sanctuary. A room that is peaceful and relaxing, and signals to your body that it's safe to shut down.

Does this sound like your room? For most people, it's not. They're paying bills in bed, working late on their laptops, scrolling their social media feeds, checking emails, or watching their favorite TV show on the flat screen hanging on the wall. We don't care about your stupid show, and newsflash—neither should you.

Stimulating activity will keep you awake. Your room should be a stress-free, device-free zone. That means no phones. No iPads. No computers. And definitely no TVs.

Energy Drain #6: Fear Dwells in the Darkness

For a lot of people struggling with insomnia, it's scary to let go of control. Sleep can make you feel vulnerable.

Just laying your head on the pillow and being in the dark with your thoughts and emotions, without distractions, can be a scary place.

Most of us know we should get to bed between 9:30 P.M. and 10:30 P.M. Yet we still go online to check the news or watch that extra episode of our favorite show.

It's like we're holding on to something or pushing it away. There's a resistance to the dark, to laying down to rest. Watch how a baby will cry and cry, fighting with every last breath against falling sleep. We're really no different, just minus the tears (or not).

Maybe it's our fear of death, of our own mortality that keeps us awake. Maybe we have some trauma in our past that catches us unaware and seemingly defenseless in the dream world. Maybe it's a fear of who we actually are when there's no more sound or anything to distract us from ourselves.

We raise these points as possibilities. We don't have the answers. Those are within you. We bring them into the light, so you can decide what's preventing you from sleeping peacefully and soundly for those eight hours.

Sometimes, it's not the answers we seek, but the questions that we ask that give us the insight we need to turn around our dis-ease.

Personal Quest (Nick)

I was in my late thirties when one morning I woke up, tried to get out of bed, and felt like I'd been beaten up in my sleep. I could barely stand, and I was in agony. I went from feeling normal to feeling like I was dying within just a couple of days.

Panicked, I called my functional medicine doc, Jay E. Williams. "I'm really scared. What do I do?" I asked.

He sent me to get a ton of blood work done, and we spent two hours going over my results. He said I had some baseline markers, but nothing out of the ordinary. Now, this is where an ordinary doctor would probably have sent me home with a shrug and maybe a prescription. But Jay asked me, "How much sleep are you getting?"

I shrugged him off. "That isn't it; I get a lot of sleep."

At that point, my oldest son was 1.5 years old. And when I really thought about it, I was getting between 5.5 and 6.5 hours a night. I thought that was pretty good, but Jay said no. This was my problem, or at least it was a big contributing factor.

He assigned me a challenge. For the next four nights, I needed to be in bed by 8:30 P.M., and I wasn't allowed to get up until I'd had eight hours.

I listened and it worked. Today I make it a priority to get in my hours most nights. It doesn't happen every night—because sometimes that's life. And if I feel my energy levels dip, my sleep is the first check-in I do.

TESTS

Beyond going in for a sleep evaluation at your local sleep center, there are some modern at-home options available to test your sleep.

Oura Ring

The Oura ring is a sleek heart-rate monitoring device that determines if you're having difficulties getting to sleep, staying asleep, or sleeping deeply. For around $300, you can have your own little sleep monitoring device wrapped around your finger.

Apple iWatch

If you don't mind the bulk of wearing your watch to bed, there are a number of apps that allow you to track your sleep on the Apple iWatch for just a few dollars. AutoSleep Tracker currently costs $2.99, and Sleep Tracker++ is $1.99. They operate very similarly to the Oura ring by running algorithms based on your heart rate levels that are measured by your watch.

THE ENERGY REMEDIES

Energy Remedy #1: Get Eight Hours of Sleep

Here's the thing about REM: we typically get there around 90 minutes after we fall asleep, and our first REM cycle is quite short—though each time we come back to it, it gets longer. For this reason, you *have* to sleep for a long enough period of time, because it's not like four hours of sleep equals four hours of REM or deep sleep.

The bottom line: you need to log at least eight hours of quality sleep. That likely means you need to start going to bed earlier. Midnight doesn't cut it for bedtime when your alarm buzzes at six.

There's an old wives' tale that says the number of hours you sleep before midnight is worth two hours for every one you log after. Research has backed this up.[11] You want the maximum number of hours available to you, so you can get in as many deep sleep cycles as possible.

If logging eight uninterrupted hours of sleep seems too much, try going to bed an hour early. Do it for three nights in one week. See how you feel.

Every little tweak to your sleeping habits can help. You owe it to yourself and your body to at least try.

Energy Remedy #2: Align with the Sun

Get thee outdoors and watch the sunset—or sunrise, if you can wake up that early. We have a friend who often asks, "Hey did you get one in?" He's talking about if you watched the sun come up or go down. If you *get one in*, that's a good day. He aims to get at least one in a day. Not only can it help reset your circadian rhythm, it can lower your stress. Let's face it, seeing the sun rise and/or set reminds us that life is beautiful, sacred, and profound. Just remembering that can relax you, and the more at peace you feel, the easier you'll drift off to slumber, while hopefully resting better too.

Energy Remedy #3:
Turn Off All Blue Lights an Hour before Bed

We're documentary filmmakers. Of course we love screens. Of course we want people to watch, learn, and love our films, and we're also very aware of how much time our culture is now hooked on electronics (we are no exception). There are so many benefits to being alive at a time as technologically advanced as today.

But when you're hooked on your devices and bathing in the blue light late into the night, you sacrifice quality sleep and your energy. Recent studies show that using screens an hour before bed can disrupt sleep.[12] Researchers have also discovered that people who use smartphones to check e-mail and do work at night are less productive and engaged the next day.[13]

You don't have to pay this price. You can get better sleep—really, you can—and you can do this without having to move to the middle of nowhere and live off the grid. But you are going to have to change some things and be proactive about your nightly routine.

It means being willing and committed to turning off your devices at least an hour or two before you go to bed, and engaging in slower, more meditative, peaceful, and restful activities. It's turning the bright lights down and maybe lighting some candles.

If you cannot part with your cell phone, then put it on airplane mode and have it at least six feet away from the bed. Don't plug it in either. This can minimize the blue light and any potential EMFs that could disrupt your sleeping. If you can, invest in a good old-fashioned alarm clock—just make sure it doesn't display a bright light.

Energy Remedy #4:
Write a To-Do List for the Next Day

There's a practice we love called the Ritual of the Moon, created by Swami Kriyananda. Every night before you go to bed, you close all the windows—meaning go to your to-do list from the day, and cross off what you finished. Next you make a to-do list for tomorrow.

The practice unburdens your mind and helps you to better manage your expectations on your time and self. Some people also keep these to-do lists on their nightstands. Right before they tuck in, they'll record all their to-dos, or if they wake up in the middle of the night, they can roll over, write it down quickly, and then fall back to sleep. It's another trick to help quiet the mind, so it's not spinning and you're not lying awake stressing about what didn't or needs to get done tomorrow.

Energy Remedy #5: Unwind and Relax

In Nick's home, his family aims to shut off the television and put their devices away between 8 P.M. and 9 P.M. After the kids are asleep, he and his wife spend an hour before bed meditating, reading, or listening to something mellow (no mainstream news scandals or horror novels that get their adrenaline pumping).

This gently calms their nervous systems from the day, so when they hit the sheets, they drift off within a few minutes and remain soundly asleep.

Energy Remedy #6: Check Your Nutrient Levels

Sometimes, what's screwing with your nervous system is actually a nutrient deficiency. You could lack B vitamins like B^6, magnesium, niacin, tryptophan, glycine, and some amino acids. Without the right equipment, your brain won't shut off.

You may need to correct the deficiency first through supplements or dietary changes, and it may take some time.

So drop the quick-fix, get-rich-in-one-night mentality that the powers that be have pushed on you. If you need to seek medical help, do it. A functional medical practitioner can test your nutrient levels, prescribe remedies, and then test them to see what works.

You don't have to go this alone.

Energy Remedy #7: Stabilize Your Blood Sugar

If you're struggling to stay asleep, then consider eating a small snack 15–20 minutes before you go to bed. "If you can stabilize your blood sugar levels right before you go to bed, it can help you have more restful sleep and also to stay asleep," explained Cassie Bjork, a registered dietician. "The key behind the bedtime snack is that it's raising blood sugar levels just a little. If you haven't eaten since dinner, which may have been a few hours ago, then your blood sugar levels are going down. If you go to bed when your blood sugar levels are on the downward cycle, it can wake you up in the middle of the night."[14]

Cassie says the best bedtime snack is fat-carbo combination. That could be a small bowl of popcorn with a little butter. A healthier choice would be half a sweet potato with a tablespoon of coconut oil or butter, or a small bowl of organic jasmine rice and steamed broccoli, or a cashew or coconut yogurt with almonds or berries, or even a small pear sautéed in a little coconut oil and topped with cinnamon and a small handful of walnuts.

Now, for all of you who are waving your arms, saying, "But it's bad to eat before going to bed!" Sure, it's bad to eat a full meal right before you go to sleep. If you're loading up and then immediately going to bed, you're probably going to gain weight and likely disrupt your sleep.

But that's not what we're talking about. We're talking about good carbs from vegetables or fruits, and healthy fats. This isn't a huge portion. It's just enough to keep your blood sugar levels in check, so you won't wake up needing a glucose hit.

Energy Remedy #8: Keep Your Bedroom Cool

Cranking the heat is a definite no-no. "As we go into the evening, our temperature naturally will start to lower," explained Dr. Stephanie Estima, a chiropractor with a special interest in functional neurology, brain optimization, and weight loss. "There are ways we can manipulate the core body temperature to help your body get cooler. One of them is your environment."[15] When the body temperature drops, it signals the brain that we're moving toward sleep, so melatonin production increases. A cool bedroom helps keep your core cool. The magic number for room temperature ranges. Some of the medical experts we spoke to suggested 65–72 degrees Fahrenheit. Others said 65–68, while the National Sleep Foundation recommends 60–67.

You may have to experiment to find the right temperature for you, but try to keep it cool rather than hot. If you need to, wear socks or a hat to bed, or use warmer blankets.

Energy Remedy #9:
Keep Your Bedroom Dark and Quiet

Any light or sound might knock you out of a deep sleep. If you haven't already, invest in blackout shades. If you have a night-light, it should be red-shifted—none of that blue light crap.

Energy Remedy #10: Cut the Coffee and Alcohol

You can love your coffee, but too much could be a bad thing. While we aren't huge coffee drinkers (we go for tea), many people are. We won't tell you to cut it entirely, but if you're a caffeine fiend *and* you sleep terribly, then try cutting back.

The effects of caffeine can last up to six hours.[16] At a minimum, try to quit by 2 P.M. If your energy is really low, then make noon your cutoff.

If you want to eliminate it entirely, then go for it. Just know that going cold turkey will probably give you nasty side effects like a massive headache. If you opt for this road, do this over the weekend. Even better, just slowly cut back until you are off caffeine. If you usually drink four cups a day, go down to three. Do this for a few days, at least, and then cut back again until the caffeine drip has turned off.

And for those wondering if they have to give up coffee forever: no way. Some of the top medical experts we spoke with said they drink coffee every day, but they do limit their intake to around two cups, and they drink it in the morning only.

Also, if you're struggling with sleep, consider how many alcoholic drinks you're enjoying every night. If it's multiple, then think about taking them out of your diet and track how you sleep. Do you sleep longer? How do you feel when you wake up? Is it easy to fall asleep? Do you wake up frequently? Once you've conquered your sleep issues, then you can add the occasional glass of your favorite beverage. Ideally, you'd drink it before, during, or right after dinner so your body has time to absorb and process the alcohol. You should also aim to stop drinking at least a couple of hours before bed.

SOLUTION

Brian started off by doing the obvious—cutting out the coffee after lunch. And it was really rough at first. He wasn't immediately sleeping any better, and so that midafternoon slump hit him hard. Without the caffeine to boost him, he struggled for a few days.

Cutting out the post-dinner coffee was a little easier. He was already exhausted, and by skipping that evening cup, he *allowed* himself to be exhausted. He opted for quiet, low-energy activities with his kids before they went to bed, like reading or just listening to them talk about their day.

After they went to bed, he wasn't allowed to crack open his laptop. Period. And honestly, he felt too tired to even try. He watched TV with his wife as usual, but he fell asleep halfway through. When he got up to brush his teeth and went to bed, his mind was still doing its racing, what-did-I-leave-undone thing, but his cell was downstairs, plugged in, and out of reach. It took him a while to fall asleep, but he did eventually, and ended up getting around five hours' sleep.

That was the first week. Once his body got used to getting a little more sleep and a lot less caffeine, he felt less tired in the afternoons and evenings. He was effective at work (and made fewer mistakes), and he was able to actually enjoy his family after work. He and his wife still had their unwind-before-the-TV routine that they enjoyed, but now they turned it off an hour or so before bed. Brian's mind still would wander before falling asleep, but he was able to get in his eight hours.

PERSONAL CHALLENGE

Try Nick's sleep challenge. For the next four nights, go to bed by 8:30, and don't get up until you've had your eight hours. Even if you don't think sleep is your issue, do it anyway. What are you going to lose? Your TV show? If something this simple can boost your energy, then hallelujah.

CHAPTER 6

Toxicity

Sandra worked hard at keeping her three kids, a husband, and a dog healthy. This meant serving them high-quality, nutritious meals (even if sometimes she had to bully her kids into eating their veggies), making sure everybody exercised (including the dog!), and keeping a clean house.

This last one was tricky, because her kids were in school and always bringing home germs. Plus, the dog tracked in things Sandra didn't want to think about too hard, so she cleaned. She scrubbed, her husband vacuumed, and she used Clorox spray bleach on all available surfaces, especially in the kitchen. She used air fresheners or scented candles, and used dryer sheets to make sure her clean laundry smelled fresh. Despite her efforts, there were occasional outbreaks of ants in the kitchen, but she sprayed as soon as she could. And of course, she always slathered sunscreen on her kids before sending them outside to play.

But no matter what she did and no matter how hard she worked, no one felt well. Most of the time her kids, her husband, and her dog were all too tired to do anything, even going for a walk. They didn't want to eat much, either—and neither did Sandra. As far as she could tell, she was doing everything right, though clearly something was going wrong.

THE PROBLEM

We can't see them, but they're everywhere. They're in our water supply, the air we breathe, the food we eat, and the millions of products we use every day.

We're talking about toxins, the elephant in the room when it comes to our exhaustion story. Of the 82,000 chemicals believed to be used in the United States, only about 25 percent have been tested.[1] Each year, the Environmental Protection Agency reviews more than 1,700 new chemical compounds.[2]

Think about that for a second. We're breathing in, slathering on, and ingesting all of these chemicals, compounds, and substances, and we have no idea what potential harm they're causing.

Modern science and medicine are starting to understand the effects chronic exposure to toxins can have on our bodies and energy levels. We know that heavy metals like mercury, lead, and aluminum can cause fatigue. Your body absorbs these toxins from simple, everyday acts like breathing in jet fuel while walking down the tarmac to an airplane or jogging on the side of the road and breathing in brake dust, or from eating sushi at your favorite restaurant.

We know that toxins can get into your cells and induce cytotoxicity, causing your cells to die. We know that toxins can impair your mitochondria. In fact, if you look at chemical research, you will find it nearly impossible to find a synthetic chemical that doesn't negatively affect mitochondrial function.

We know that toxins can lead to a sluggish gallbladder and slow the production of bile, which can impair your liver—the king detox organ of your body. We know that a toxin found in herbicides, called *glyphosate*, can affect your gut, specifically a protein called *zonulin*, which makes your gut lining more permeable, leading to leaky gut. And almost every physician we spoke with said they have treated patients suffering from exhaustion caused by toxins, though their patients had no idea toxicity was even a thing.

That's why we call this the elephant in the room when we talk about exhaustion. It's becoming a bigger cause for why people are so damn tired, but modern science and medicine are just beginning to talk more about it, which is wild. We've known the dangers of toxins and chemicals since Rachel Carson brought the destructive effects of DDT to the attention of the public in her seminal work, *Silent Spring,* published in 1962. Six decades later, we're still coming to terms with and awakening to the realization that toxicity exists.

People today get that pesticides are a thing. They get that genetically modified food is a thing. But hidden toxins in their soap, in their perfume, in their clothing, and in their plastic water bottles that could be wrecking their health and causing them to be painfully exhausted?

"There's this whole issue of toxic overload that's much more subtle, harder to track. But it's real," said Dr. Robert Rountree, an integrative practitioner who combines traditional family medicine, nutrition, medical herbology, and mind-body therapy. "Patients come in saying, 'I'm tired.' Normally, I would tell them 'take a nap,' but it's not that easy. They go to sleep and wake up, and they're still tired. Something else must be going on, and I think toxicity is a good bet for a lot of people."[3]

If you've gotten this far in the book, if you've tried many of the remedies and nothing is working, then it's worth considering whether you have a toxic overload.

We realize this chapter may seem scary, but we promise you that this is not doom and gloom. We're going to show you where some of these toxins may be hiding before explaining how they could be affecting your liver, immune system, and mitochondria, causing you to lose energy.

This chapter is all about awareness. It's about helping you make the best choices about what you put in, put on, and expose your body to. We'll always have toxins in our environment. That's the world we live in today. We can't avoid them, and we can't walk around in hazmat suits either.

But we *can* manage our exposure. We *can* make small tweaks to our daily lives so we can tip the scales back in our favor. The remedies in this chapter will help you do just that—make some simple adjustments to start evening the score against these invaders.

Still, we want to be straight with you. If your energy levels were knocked out due to a toxin, especially a heavy metal like lead, mercury, or aluminum, you need to see a doctor. We're going to recommend various tests that will indicate if you've got heavy metals in your system—if you think that's a remote possibility, you should definitely get yourself tested.

The modern era needs modern solutions. Hopefully, your doctor runs a toxin panel and says, "Nothing to see here, you're fine," and that's great. Go, move on, and find the real root for your exhaustion, crossing off toxicity as one less thing to worry about.

But if your body is lit up with toxins, you're not going to feel better until you get that poison out of your system, which isn't something you can do at home. The good news is you *can* beat them. We've seen other people do it, and we know how amazing people feel after they get their toxin issue under control. It may take a little detective work, it may mean going to a doctor who specializes in treating heavy metals or other toxins, but it's totally doable.

In this chapter, stay objective. Stay rational. Stay focused on beating back your exhaustion—you can do it.

THE ENERGY DRAINS

Energy Drain #1:
Hidden Toxins Are Catching You Unaware

If we're exposed to 47,000 toxins every year, where are they coming from? Simply put, everywhere. It's such an exhaustive list that it can get overwhelming.

That's why we're highlighting some of the major areas where you're likely to find them. This is all about raising your awareness, so you can make different choices about what products, environments, foods, and other modern-day conveniences you're exposed to.

Now, we understand that you don't always have choices. If you live in Chicago or Los Angeles, or downstream from a coal mine in West Virginia, you get what you get. If you see something on this list that isn't in your control, don't get discouraged. Just focus on what is in your control. It will still make a difference.

Air

We have never had so many particulates in the air as we do today. If you're in an urban environment, you could be getting jet fuel, kerosene, particulate matter from car exhaust. Polycyclic aromatic hydrocarbons (PAHs), by-products from burning fossil fuels, have been shown to increase the likelihood of learning and behavior disorders in children. High prenatal exposure to PAHs are associated with attention issues, anxiety, and depression in children.[4]

But want to know where the dirtiest air is? The answer may actually surprise you—it's in your home. Toxins waft into your air from plug-in air fresheners, scented candles, from the cleaning products you use. You also have carpets and furniture like your couch, possibly your mattress, that are treated with flame-retardants. That may seem like a good thing, but it also can release the chemical bromine, which can irritate the respiratory tract.[5] Flame-retardant mattresses may also release carbon monoxide, which we all know can kill us in large doses.

The *American Journal of Respiratory and Critical Care Medicine* says that regular use of air freshener sprays can increase your risk of developing asthma by as much as 50 percent. Air fresheners contain phthalates, which are also found in perfumes, as sealants in adhesives, and tons of other places. Phthalates can cause reproductive, endocrine, and developmental issues—and phthalates are often not listed among the ingredients, even when the brand is labeled "all-natural" or "unscented."

Air fresheners also emit terpene, which reacts with the air around you to create formaldehyde . . . which is, you know, not great.

Some candles, including unscented ones, can contain paraffin, a sludge waste product of petroleum. When we burn paraffin, we release carcinogenic chemicals. Now, we're not saying you can't burn candles, just make sure they're good ones. Soy and beeswax candles are perfectly safe.

Polluting your air makes it hard to breathe, and when you can't breathe, you don't have the oxygen your body needs to make it go and do things. It's that simple.

Food

We know that organic farming practices tend to be healthier than conventional practices.

We also know that eating whole, natural food is better. Mother Nature provides us with everything we need to sustain our bodies.

But in humankind's quest for unlimited supplies and growth, we've nuked our plants with harmful pesticides and destroyed our soils. We've injected our animals with growth hormones and antibiotics. We've created addictive foods loaded with chemical additives and preservatives. There's just way too much to list—you'd go blind trying to read the chemical names alone.

What are these pesticides and chemicals doing to us? Well, sadly, this hasn't been studied all that closely (for reasons that paranoid people like us think have to do with lobbying and an intentional lack of government oversight). But in Sweden, scientists measured the toxic intake of organic foods versus regular foods and found that people had a 70 percent lower exposure to toxins just from eating organic.[6]

And, bonus—eating organic is actually *good* for you. You get more antioxidants, more omega-3s, more flavonols, not to mention better flavor, when you eat organic.[7]

Personal Care Products

"What you put on your body, you put *in* your body," said Dani Williamson, an integrative health-care nurse practitioner. "Whatever you're putting on your body, you want to make sure it's clean, nontoxic, and anti-inflammatory because it's a piece of the puzzle."[8] If you're not looking at your skincare ingredients, you could be slathering on sludge and giving yourself a really big hole to dig out from. This can include skincare, haircare, sunscreen, and cosmetics. Under current law, cosmetic companies do not have to conduct safety assessments on their products, which places consumers at greater risk for possible exposure.

Some of the toxins found in these products may include:

Phthalates, which are a group of chemicals that may disrupt the endocrine system, which is responsible for hormone production. (You'll remember these from air fresheners.) This can interfere with development, reproductive, and neurological damage. You won't see this listed in the ingredient list. It can just be called "fragrance." Phthalates could be found in deodorant, scented lip balm, or nail polish.

Polyethylene glycols, or PEGs, are petroleum-based compounds used in cream-based products. These compounds are often contaminated with ethylene oxide, a known human carcinogen, potentially harmful to the nervous system and human development.

Butylated compounds (BHT, BHA). These are endocrine disruptors, like phthalates, which may cause skin allergies, and are linked to organ, developmental, and reproductive toxicity. These compounds are used as preservatives and may be found in eyeliners, eye shadows, lip glosses, perfumes (even in food like chips, beer, baked goods, vegetable oil, and chewing gum).

The list of personal care products includes lotions, shampoos, makeup, shaving creams, sunscreens, and so many more, so you do have to watch out.

One of the challenges with our products is we don't feel or notice any immediate effects. We're getting microdoses of toxins with each application that add up over time, slowly damaging our systems in the long run. Take lipstick. Who would ever swallow a tube of lipstick? No one. But as a woman goes about her day, maybe reapplying it a few times, where does that lipstick eventually go? Right down the hatch. And if you do that for 10 years, that gunk can add up in your system, especially when you consider the number of products you're ingesting or absorbing right along with it.

Deodorant is another example. We may be doing ourselves and the people around us a favor by keeping body odor to a minimum, but if we're not careful, we could be dosing ourselves with aluminum (which has possible links to cancer and Alzheimer's). Thankfully, there are many aluminum-free choices on the market today, but it does take some hunting to find the right products. Schmidt's is a good choice, or you can even search for "homemade deodorant" to find a recipe for a healthy homemade version.

The good news is that finding the right products is much easier today than ever. Even if you live in a rural area, you can buy healthier products online. If you're in a larger metropolis, check out local health food stores, big and small.

A great first step away from the toxic sludge is to look for natural ingredients. Rule of thumb—only buy products with ingredients that you can pronounce and recognize. Also, consider buying organic, but read the label carefully. Up to 5 percent of ingredients are allowed to be from nonorganic sources. Look for 100 percent organic.

Household Goods

Do you use plastic wrap to cover and reheat food in the microwave? That plastic contains chemicals, including phthalates. The steam melts the plastic, which drips the toxins into your food. You want to ditch the plastic wrap.

Also, check out your containers. Are they glass or plastic? Hopefully, glass. Plastic can contain BPA, which is bisphenol A, an industrial chemical used to make certain plastics. It has been linked to fertility and reproductive issues, heart disease, and many other conditions.[9]

Cleaning supplies contain volatile chemicals like chlorine, ammonia, sodium hydroxide, and more. These can be so damaging that in Los Angeles, these chemicals are creating more smog than the area's more regulated cars.[10]

Polytetrafluoroethylene, the coating that makes your pan "nonstick," releases gases when heated—gases that have been shown to be carcinogenic.

Flea and tick treatments for your pet are pesticides. This may seem obvious, but is it something you think about when you scratch Achilles on the back of his neck and then touch your face?

Mycotoxins/Mold

A lot of people believe black mold only happens in wet climates like the deep south. It's really everywhere. Even in Boulder where it's dry as hell, there's a ridiculous amount of black mold that makes people sick.

We have a few friends who were suffering from terrible fatigue, and it came down to a substantial mold exposure. This is one of those toxin categories that many people refuse to take seriously, but trust us—airborne mold ain't fiction. It can silently destroy your life.

If you're sucking on fumes with your energy, then it may be worth checking out your mold situation, including your water heater.

Dental Fillings

About 50 percent of amalgam dental fillings are mercury.[11] They're supposedly stable. Keyword, "supposedly." For some people, their fillings are releasing tiny mercury particles that get swallowed every day. If you have an amalgam filling, it's not as simple as sprinting to the dentist and asking him to remove it and replace it with porcelain either. If the fillings get removed, the drill can vaporize the filling, which can cause the mercury to leak into their systems.

If you have mercury fillings, you'll want to seek guidance from a professional before you take any major action.

Pharmaceutical Drugs

We live in a culture where modern, Western medicine is all about alleviating symptoms with drugs. If you're not feeling well, as a well-intentioned patient, you go to your doctor, who says, "Here, take this pill."

You do and maybe they've made a few symptoms go away, but now you don't have any energy to hang with your family and kids, you can't sleep with your mate, and life starts spiraling down because you're struggling to get through the day.

The difference between medicine and poison is dose. There may be nothing wrong with your prescriptions, but they may affect your body in subtle ways that drain your energy and could make your body toxic too.

EMFs

We don't know exactly what's going on with all of these electromagnetic frequencies and blue lights. The research and data aren't in yet, so we don't know the fallout.

But we do know that people have anecdotally reported they feel better when they shut off their Wi-Fi at night and when they remove their cell phones and other electronics from their nightstands. It could be the mental or emotional relief that can come from turning off our devices and giving ourselves a break.

While we can't in good faith tell you what 4G and 5G are doing to your body, if you're struggling to find the root of your exhaustion, and nothing is working, then try reducing your EMF exposure.

It certainly won't hurt you.

Toxic Relationships

People can poison us. They can draw upon our energy, leaving us exhausted. We're going to talk more about how relationships and energy vampires can affect our energy levels in Chapter 9. For now, just be aware that the people surrounding you could be the source of your toxicity.

Energy Drain #2: Your Liver Is Overwhelmed

"We are all toxic, but it's a matter of how toxic are you and how toxic am I, and how well does your body work getting rid of toxins," said Dr. Afrouz Demeri, naturopathic doctor specializing in hormonal imbalance. "The main organ that is the most important for energy and toxins is the liver."[12]

Our bodies are designed to eliminate toxins as they come into the body. But this was before we humans trashed the planet and began bathing ourselves in synthetics. In our world today, these toxins build up, and if your liver can't keep up, you're in trouble—and likely exhausted.

Your liver is the star player in detoxing your body. Technically, the liver is a gland, and it is responsible for over 500 jobs in your body. The liver has multiple jobs. One of its jobs—we'll call it the day job—is to take glucose from the food you've eaten and digested, and store it as glycogen to help you manage your energy throughout the day. It will also draw on these glycogen reserves at night so the brain gets all the energy it needs for its brainwash.

One of the liver's other jobs—we'll call it a night job—is to detox your system. It filters blood coming from the digestive system before sending it off to the rest of the body, clearing out toxins and chemicals, including pharmaceuticals, alcohol, and all that stuff we mentioned in Energy Drain #1.

It does this in two phases. In Phase One, it uses oxidation. We think of oxidation as being bad—it's the deterioration of cells. But, in this case, oxidation is being used for a good cause, as the liver breaks down toxins that are typically fat soluble, and makes them water soluble and therefore easier to eliminate.

Simple, right? Well, not necessarily. Sometimes those water-soluble toxins are actually worse for you than when they were fat soluble, and so they need to be broken down further.

Enter Phase Two. Now we perform conjugation, in which these toxins are paired with other substances, including sulfur and certain amino acids, so that they can then be expelled along with bile (which your liver excretes for normal digestive function).

Cool. But it's really easy for the liver to get overwhelmed, particularly if it gets bogged down in Phase One. The liver can barely do its own job in this day and age. When you start putting artificial hormones or hormone-like derivatives in your food, in your shampoos, in your personal care products, that all needs to get conjugated by the liver. Then when you add diesel truck fumes and the thousands of other toxins you're exposed to, your liver simply cannot handle it.

If your boss kept throwing a bunch of files onto your desk, demanding you work under unreasonable deadlines, and this went on year after year, you'd burn out and probably want to quit. This is how your liver feels as more and more toxins build up.

The liver still has its day job, storing glucose, which also starts to suffer. Very quickly, the liver gets overwhelmed with more glucose than it needs for storage, but it still has to stash the glucose somewhere. That somewhere is as fat.

This is why you hear about intentional detoxes with herbs, special diets, lots of water, even fasting. Each tool is designed to help the liver detox and function more efficiently. When your liver is firing on all cylinders, your system can handle many demands placed on it.

We know detoxing may seem intimidating, so we've included a simple how-to-get-started primer in the Remedies section.

Energy Drain #3:
Your Immune System Has Been Invaded

Our world is so toxic that our immune systems are becoming overwhelmed.

It begins as soon as we're born. In an Environmental Working Group study of newborns, researchers found an average of 200 different industrial chemicals and pollutants in the umbilical cords of newborns.[13] These weren't mild toxins, either. Out of the 287 toxic substances, 180 were carcinogenic, 217 were toxic to the brain and nervous system, and 208 can cause developmental problems.[14]

Since the Industrial Revolution, it's gotten worse. Five hundred years ago, the list of chemicals could fit into one long paragraph.[15] Today, we have created over 150 million chemicals that are in use in every product, on every surface, in every material we use.[16] That number has tripled in just 25 years. In 1975, we only had 50 million chemicals.[17] *Only.*

It's a huge dumpster fire that your immune system doesn't know how to put out. For millions of years, your immune system was trained to recognize and familiarize itself with the trees, plants, animals, air, water, rocks, and other things found in your native environment.

Nick's ancestors came from Italy, so his system understands the environmental compounds from that region. Pedram's family came from Iran, so his system understands what's found in Iran.

The world's become mobile. Both of us have transplanted to the Rockies. Our immune systems now are like "What the hell is this? Is it friend or foe?" They've had to adjust quickly to a new territory.

Our bodies are pretty resilient. When exposed to stuff like pollen that comes from nature, our immune systems will go "friend or foe?" and mostly they can figure out what to let in and what to keep out.

But you start adding stuff like arsenic, Italian perfume, and all of these synthetically manufactured substances in a lab, and the body doesn't know what on earth to do with it. It doesn't even recognize half of it.

It's like having a UFO land on Main Street, USA. Everyone would freak out—justifiably. To make it worse, it's not just one UFO; you have a damn fleet arriving in your immune system. Every. Single. Day.

These substances, these chemicals and compounds that you eat, drink, put on, or breath in, are seriously alien in origin. If they were synthesized in a lab, *maybe* they resemble something the body once could have recognized in nature, but they're still "new." Your body doesn't know what to do with "new." It wasn't trained for this.

These UFOs land, and your body goes into DEFCON 3, red alert, man your battle stations. The only way it knows to defend itself is to mount an immune response, launching IgA antibodies to track and destroy the invaders. That alone will make you tired, but hopefully it'll get the job done.

If it doesn't get the job done (like say you're exposed to heavy metals like mercury or aluminum or something the body can't identify), not only will you be tired, but your immune system has to go into "operation: capture and contain the threat."

You can't just have toxins in free-flow circulation, so your body shunts them away in your *fat*. Your body signals to your thyroid to slow down and start making fat, so the body can jail the intruders.

You probably see where we're going with this. One day, you look in the mirror and decide you want to lose extra pounds, so you start working out. Theoretically, losing weight and burning that fat as fuel would be a good thing. Not so when your fat is storing those toxins.

When you break down that body fat, you then release toxins from their cage. Now they're back in your bloodstream, and you've unintentionally poisoned yourself. Your immune system is like, "Dude, I thought we took care of this? Get them back in their cages." The body goes and makes more fat to store toxins, essentially saying, "just be fat; it's safer for you."

It's the ultimate "screw you" to weight loss and yo-yo weight gain, and a major reason why we have an obesity epidemic in America. Our bodies are way more toxic than we're talking about, or willing to, and until some people address their toxicity issue, they'll never burn that fat as fuel.

That fat, the fat we're all so busy hating, is actually the thing keeping us alive. It's sequestering the toxins and chemicals and substances that could seriously harm you.

In this story, *fat is your hero*. How wild is that? It sure makes us see our body fat in a different light.

Energy Drain #4:
Your Mitochondria Have Bitten the Dust

Dr. Tom O'Bryan, an expert in food sensitivities, environmental toxins, and the development of autoimmune diseases, uses an example
that we love. Imagine you just woke up, and you're dragging. It's
already been a long week—it's Tuesday—so you hit up Starbucks on
your way to work for your daily caffeine fix.

The baristas stick a plastic cap on your cup so you don't spill
hot coffee and burn yourself. Of course, you don't think anything
of it. You just sip happily away, now alert and ready to power
through your day.

But that plastic cap is probably made with BPA, and when the
hot steam wafts up from the cup, it melts the plastic cap so that now
the BPA drips into your coffee. Every sip you take that you think is
energizing you is actually setting you back because BPA shuts down
your mitochondria.

Mitochondria have shown themselves to be the canary in the
coal mine when it comes to toxin exposures. A number of toxins
such as heavy metals, BPA, and fluoride have been found to damage
your mitochondria, in the worst case shutting them down and killing them off.

No mitochondria mean no energy producers and no defenders
for your cells. That's trouble. This leaves you more exhausted and
more susceptible to threats. If you're low on mitochondria, your
immune system can't do its job killing off the invaders.

It's not just that your mitochondria die off. As we talked about
in Chapter 3, when toxins invade your system and cause an immune
system response, it signals to your mitochondria to shut down
energy production and get ready to defend the cells. The more your
mitochondria stay in defense mode, the less time they spend producing energy, so the exhaustion just amps up.

Energy Drain #5: You're Drinking from the Tap

New York City has one of the best marketing strategies ever. The
city government even markets its tap water as some of the best
anywhere. "New York City drinking water is world-renowned for

its quality," reads its website.[18] They rave about how it's from clean reservoirs in the Catskill Mountains, and how "The Department of Environmental Protection performs more than 900 tests daily, 27,000 monthly, and 330,000 on an annual basis from up to 1,200 sampling locations throughout New York City."

Don't get us wrong, that's impressive, and you sure as hell want your water supply tested so it's not swimming with *E. coli*, giardia, legionella. But come visit the Rocky Mountains, drink some natural spring water, then go back to New York City and take a sip. It's like drinking pool water. It's got chlorine. It's got fluoride. It's got disinfectant. It's got this metallic, tin taste.

It's not just New York City with this problem—it's everywhere in America. Rural, suburban, and urban.

Most people think what flows from their tap is completely safe. Well, it's often not. Sure, we've largely removed the big baddies that our water quality experts know to look for, but we've also doused our water with crazy amounts of chemicals to exterminate the bugs.

It's like we're back in 2002, before the organic food movement became a household phrase. Our water quality issues are so under the radar that most people have no idea just how toxic their H_2O is.

For example, there's fluoride, which is added to tap water in every state (though the top 10 in terms of percentage are Kentucky, Minnesota, Illinois, Maryland, North Dakota, Georgia, Virginia, Indiana, South Carolina, and South Dakota).[19] When it was introduced in the 1940s, it was hailed as an enormous breakthrough in public health helping to prevent tooth decay.[20] And yeah, fluoride makes your teeth stronger, but recent studies have found that in high enough doses, it can damage your bones and joints, cause neurological disorders, and impact your thyroid along with a whole host of other problems.[21] If you're drinking a lot of tap water, or brushing your teeth and using a mouthwash (both with fluoride), your levels may be too high.

It's unlikely you'll get sick overnight and die after drinking from your tap, but ingesting all that fluoride, along with BPA, disinfectants, or pesticide residues (all of which are found in public water) accumulates year after year.

We've all heard about Flint, Michigan, and other communities with severe lead poisoning in the water. Health impacts, particularly on children, can include impaired cognition, hearing problems, behavioral disorders, and delayed puberty.

We're not throwing stones at our public water supply officials or the idea of purifying water supplies. There are major diseases that can lurk in water. You get cholera, you can die.

But we are just starting to understand the real story and the unintended consequences like exhaustion that have come from the accumulation of water treatment products in our system over many years.

Personal Quest (Pedram)

I grew up in Southern California. My family moved down to the Huntington Beach area, and it's pretty great down there. We drank filtered water, but we figured, this is California. We can probably cook with the tap water. It's not like we're going to get cholera or anything.

But what we didn't think about is how there were oil wells off the coast about 50 years ago. I did my tox profile, and my aluminum and uranium levels were high. Turns out if you spend a decade cooking with that shit, it's not great. I was just mainlining uranium every time I boiled pasta.

Uranium sounds scary—and it is—but fortunately we're not talking about the radioactive stuff. But still, this is in clean metropolitan groundwater. I got it out of my system, and I installed a reverse osmosis filter under the sink so we wouldn't cook with it anymore. Six months later, I retested, and my levels were fine.

Lesson learned: don't just detox; fix the source of the problem.

TESTS

Another big piece may be working with a professional to find out how toxic your body is. If you're really struggling to lose weight or your energy is just so low you can barely function and you've tried everything up to this point, then it could be a toxicity issue. If it is, then you need the help of a professional, likely beyond your general practitioner, to get your levels in a normal range.

We do have to warn you, these tests can get expensive. You'll want to work with an expert who will really listen to your symptoms first, and who asks lots of questions about your lifestyle and where you live. This will help them narrow down the most likely culprits to test for. For example, if you eat sushi for lunch every day, they may want to test your mercury levels.

What are some tests they may run? Let's check them out.

Blood Test

Your doctor can measure a lot of different toxins that are swimming in your blood stream. We're talking heavy metals like aluminum, mercury, arsenic, barium, lead, tin, zinc, and many more.

Urine Challenge

Blood tests will tell you what's in your bloodstream at the moment—so whatever you've recently digested, but hasn't been stored in your body yet. A urine challenge will go a lot deeper. First, you get a urine test, again to determine your normal background levels, and then you take something called DMSA, DMPS, or EDTA—this will juice your cells, drawing out all the crap you've got stored in them.

Over a six-hour collection period, you will catch all your pee in a bucket, basically, and then send it into the lab, where they'll see what you're really carting around. This is the gold standard of toxicity tests, and it is definitely something you need to do with a doctor.

THE ENERGY REMEDIES

Energy Remedy #1: Reduce Your Toxin Exposure

We live in a highly toxic world. You can't become bubble boy or girl and expect to eliminate all threats. But you can become more aware of the conscious choices you're making, and what you're surrounding your body with and putting into and onto it. You'll never get rid of all the toxins in and around you, but getting rid of *some* can be game changing.

To do this, first you need some awareness on your exposure levels and what you're being exposed to. This is all about stacking the odds in your favor as much as you can.

Here are some of our best picks for reducing your toxic load.

Use a Home Air Filter

We can't do much about exhaust from diesel trucks driving by, but we can prevent it from smogging up our homes. Here are some options:

- If allergens are an issue: the Coway Mighty Air Purifier eliminates particles—including pollen and allergens—as small as .3 microns.

- If you're concerned about mold: GermGuardian Elite 3-in-1 has antimicrobial agents and UVC lights to kill mold and germs.

- If you're in a smoky environment: Oransi Max can clear gas particles.

Open Your Windows

If you're more concerned about getting rid of toxins that are inside your house than in getting rid of those coming in from outside—open your windows! Let that fresh air come in.

Eat Organic

This is not earth-shattering news. We know conventional produce is sprayed with all sorts of chemicals and toxins. Research conducted by UC Berkeley School of Public Health found that families eating a completely organic diet for one week reduced traces of pesticides in their system by an average of 60 percent.[22]

Switch Personal Care Products

Personal care products are one of the biggest culprits when it comes to toxins, so the next time you're out, try looking for ones that are 100 percent organic and free of parabens. Read the labels on your makeup, deodorant, shampoo, soap, and everything you're putting on your body. Go as natural as possible. If you feel overwhelmed with choices, then consider checking out sites that have done some of the work for you like the Environmental Working Group (ewg.org/skindeep). Their site allows you to search by brand, ingredients, or products to find safer personal care products.

Energy Remedy #2: Try a Detox

Detoxing is not a new thing. It's been going on for thousands of years, and people have known and benefited from it.

Our ancestors have been considering detoxing for centuries. Nick works closely with K. P. Khalsa, one of the foremost natural healing experts in North America, who talks about how when you detox, you're not just detoxing from the toxins you've picked up in the environment, but the toxins passed down through generations.

We know this may sound a little far out there, and we're not saying we're believers. But the belief in detoxing and the need to remove the impurities from our bodies is something that we as human beings have carried with us for a very long time.

Intentionally detoxing our bodies is just as important, perhaps even more so, today. "We live in a very toxic world, no doubt," explained Dr. David Perlmutter. "It's a world unlike anything that has confronted our ancestors. We have not evolved the detoxification safeguards to allow us to deal with all the toxins to which we are exposed, so we need to do our best to augment our detoxification pathways. When we understand how to do that, we can give ourselves a leg up to deal with some of the toxic exposures we have."[23]

To help prime your detoxing pathways, here are the most common techniques (you've probably heard of at least some of them):

Clean, Raw, or Alkaline Cleanses

These are all basically the same and consist of focusing on eating raw plants—so fruits, vegetables, raw nuts, seeds, and sprouts. The idea here is to get you a ton of phytonutrients, micronutrients, fiber, and enzymes that might otherwise be denatured through cooking, thereby cleaning out your liver, colon, and kidneys, as well as your lungs and skin. If your blood levels are overly acidic, then these detoxes can help balance your pH. These cleanses take about a month.

Master Cleanse

We probably all know somebody who has done this. It's when you combine fresh lemon juice, cayenne pepper, Grade B maple syrup, and water. For a bonus, you can add some psyllium husks. Either way, you're going to poop a lot. You can do this for 3–10 days. You drop weight like crazy, and you clear out a ton of toxins.

Liquid, Juice Cleanse

This is just what it sounds like. Lots and lots of water, along with fresh organic vegetable juices, liquid soups like miso, and green or berry smoothies. You want to focus on dark, leafy greens like parsley, basil, celery, cabbage, cilantro, and cucumber, as well as carrots, beets, ginger, and turmeric. This can be done over 3 days, or for up to 2 weeks.

Now, some words of caution: just like with fasting, be smart about this. Pay attention to your body's response. Cleansing is great *if you do it right*. Because you're eating so few foods, your body tends to focus in on them pretty severely, so what you eat will have an outsize impact. This means it is more important than ever to eat organic.

This is pretty obvious, since we're getting rid of toxins here, but it really matters. Your body is trying to clear out toxins, and it's using every bit of food it gets. Make sure you're giving it the good stuff.

Also, just because something is good for a little while doesn't mean it's good for the long term. You need to eat food, okay? Don't keep going with your cayenne and lemon juice and think that's going to be good for your long-term survival. You can do yourself a lot of harm if you go overboard.

You can absolutely detox too much, and if you're using it to cover up unhealthy lifestyle choices, you could do more harm than good. In L.A., the new word for dieting is detox. If you're out partying and eating a bunch of tacos at 4:30 A.M., still gargling tequila, and thinking, *eh, I'm detoxing in three days, no biggie*, you've got other changes you need to make.

Once you've done a detox, get back to healthy eating habits.

Energy Remedy #3:
Add More Natural Detoxing to Your Daily Life

Sometimes, you don't need a huge detox program. Just adding more tools to your daily life can help your body and energy levels. We've included a few areas for you to experiment with.

Try adding a few to the daily swings and see what happens.

Eat Some Salsa

Onions, garlic, and cilantro squeeze out the heavy metals from your cells, so just eat salsa all the time! You'll need to monitor your chip intake, though.

Sweat It Out

Put on some sweatpants and get to work. Your liver and your kidneys are your primary detox organs, but whatever they can't handle gets squeezed out through the skin in your sweat.

Here's an at-home workout to get you sweating. Set a timer and do the following:

- 5 pushups (do them on your knees, against a wall, or another inclined surface, if necessary)
- 20 crunches
- 20 jumping jacks
- 10 squats

Your goal is to move for about 10 minutes. You want to kick up your heart rate, and to get some sweat on the brow. One round may do the trick for you or you may need to do more. Listen to your body. You want to sweat and breath heavy, but you shouldn't be light-headed or gasping for air. If you are, back off the intensity. Conversely, you want to sweat, so if it's too easy, pick up the pace or up those numbers.

And if you're feeling flat-on-your-back exhausted, skip this entirely! Remember, meet yourself where you're at, and wherever that is, it's exactly where you need to be.

And for the days when you're just not up to moving it enough to sweat, that's okay. Treat yourself to an *infrared sauna*. Yeah, this is pretty bougie, and we're not suggesting you go out and buy one, but 20–30 minutes sweating in a sauna can help you release those toxins.

Eat More Bitters

Look around at different cultures and you'll see most traditionally have a before-dinner drink. Traditionally, most of these drinks have been bitter. Even beer is bitter. Bitters prime our digestion to produce the juices we need to break down our food. The more you're breaking down your food, the easier it is for the liver to work its magic.

By adding more bitters to your diet, you're helping your liver detox.

Bitter could mean any bitter vegetable, including cruciferous ones like broccoli, kale, cauliflower, broccoli sprouts, and radishes. Add three to four cups of these vegetables, preferably cooked, to your diet every day, or try swapping your romaine lettuce for arugula, which is a bitter.

Try Supplements and Herbs

The most popular supplement is *milk thistle*, which helps the liver cleanse itself of toxins. Sulfur amino acids like methyl donors, and SAMe, and methionine can also be very effective. Even supplements like vitamins C and B can help the liver.

Drink Plenty of Water

There are some really weird detoxes online, involving pills and juices and whatnot—don't fall prey to any old salesperson schilling the latest and greatest gimmick.

Just staying hydrated and drinking filtered water can do wonders for your liver and your kidneys. Water flushes your system, so drink up.

Energy Remedy #4: Get Those Mitochondria in Shape

As mentioned before, the best thing you can do for your mitochondria is to promote mitophagy. Urolithin A, found in pomegranates and in supplement form, can clear out your old mitochondria, making room for the new.

You should also make sure to eat plenty of antioxidants to offset cellular damage in the first place, especially glutathione, an amino acid that protects your mitochondria. (Bonus: it also detoxifies.)[24] It is available as a supplement, but you can also boost levels by choosing foods high in its precursor nutrients, including garlic, onion, cruciferous vegetables like broccoli, cauliflower, cabbage, and brussels sprouts, as well as asparagus, peppers, carrots, avocados, squash, and spinach.

And, as ever, make sure you're getting plenty of magnesium.

Energy Remedy #5: Clean Your Water

City water often isn't all that great. Essentially, more pavement means less water soaking into the ground, which means that the water table will have less new water coming in to recharge it. Instead, excess rain forms runoff, which is funneled through drains into streams . . . which frequently also contain sewage and industrial waste. Water tends to be cleaner outside of cities.[25]

But no matter where you are, there are contaminants, and you should spend the time and money working to clear them out as much as possible.

We're in favor of still having a planet to live on, so we're not advocating buying bottled water all the time. Instead, buy *a water filter* for your home that can pull out many chemicals from the tap. You can get these filters for your kitchen faucet and just screw it on to the tap. You can get them for your water tank as well. The doctors we spoke with said water filters are an absolute must if you use city water.

Here are two of our favorites:

- The iSpring RC77 5-Stage rests under your sink, so your water comes out already filtered. It uses reverse osmosis to get rid of 99.9% of harmful contaminants.

- The Apex MR-1050 sits on your sink, and uses an alkaline filter, which means that you receive minerals like calcium, magnesium, and potassium, which is a nice bonus. This filter also balances the pH of your water.

SOLUTION

Sandra wasn't wrong about wanting to keep a clean house—we all want that, even if some of us have a hard time achieving it. We give Sandra so much credit.

And yet, Sandra's urge to clean was impacting the health of her family. In her concern about germs, she was using chlorine bleach all over the house, even in places where food was prepared. Now there's not a ton of chlorine in these sprays, certainly not enough to send someone to the hospital for chlorine poisoning (unless her kids drank it or something), but there is enough to make you feel off—even exhausted.

It took Sandra a little while to realize what was going on, but she figured it out when she got a little of the stuff in her eyes. If the spray felt like *that*, what was it doing to her insides, when she ingested it along with her food?

She switched to a homemade cleaning spray using white vinegar, water, and essential oils. White vinegar is acetic acid and serves as a great disinfectant—it can tackle salmonella, *E. coli*, and other bacteria.

It was a simple fix, and it saved her some money. And soon enough, Sandra and her family were back up and running.

PERSONAL CHALLENGE

We know we're supposed to drink eight glasses of water a day, but do any of us really do that? We challenge you to test yourself. Eight glasses of water are a half gallon. Get a half-gallon jug and fill it with filtered water, and see if you can drink the whole thing in one day.

Keep going, every day for a week. At first it might seem like way too much, but you'll find that your body will get used to it—even start to crave it. Give it a try, and see how you feel.

CHAPTER 7

Adrenals and Hormones

Bethany leads a very hectic, high-powered career in advertising.

A typical day has her drinking six to eight cups of coffee (sometimes more!), running on very little sleep, responding to emails and client requests at night and on the weekends, and attending lots of client dinners and conferences. She's achieved a certain degree of career success, for sure, but it seems to have come at a price.

For the last three years, Bethany has tried to get pregnant.

She's seen all the specialists. She's changed her diet and taken different drugs that have messed with her hormones and caused wild mood swings. She's even dealing with adult acne, insomnia, no sex drive, and she's tired all the time.

At wit's end, she and her husband are considering spending $30,000 on IVF therapy. She'll do it, but she can't help feeling like a failure. Struggling to get pregnant has really challenged her sense of self and identity as a woman. "Normal" women can conceive, she tells herself. Her sister and many of her friends did so without any problems. For some reason, she's stuck.

Most of her doctors have been dismissive about her struggles, which makes her feel even more like a failure.

Now in her early 40s, getting pregnant has become deeply personal for Bethany. She's scared she's running out of time to conceive and give birth naturally. She's at a point where she needs to have a child now or give up the idea of it. She really doesn't want to give up, but with no sex drive and no energy, she doesn't know where to go.

THE PROBLEM

Hormones.

A lot of people think of hormones as something that happened to them when they were 13, or when they're trying to have a baby. But when you start understanding what hormones actually do in your body, you realize, they are a *big deal*.

Hormones are essentially chemical messengers that pass orders between your organs and cells. Often, it's information that doesn't even go through your brain.

We already talked about when there's glucose in your bloodstream, it signals to your pancreas to create and release the hormone insulin. That insulin is a messenger that travels to your cells, knocking on their front door saying, "Hey, open up, we've got a delivery of glucose coming for the mitochondria to turn into energy."

Your brain wasn't involved in that. It happened as naturally as you breathe.

Every day your body creates and releases hundreds of hormones from glands such as the pituitary, pineal, thyroid, pancreas, testicles, ovaries, thymus, and adrenals. These glands make up our *endocrine system*. The endocrine system is an information highway that allows our cells, organs, and bodies as a whole to communicate with each other seamlessly.

Our challenge today is that our modern world and lifestyle can scramble these messengers, and when our hormones aren't working right, then our organs, cells, and bodies don't work right. And when our bodies aren't working right, energy can't be produced properly and we can end up exhausted.

Our aim in this chapter is to help you better understand what might be happening with your hormone levels. We're focusing on your adrenal glands, which play a huge role in regulating your energy, sleep, immune system, and metabolism. We're also going to walk you through what happens when hormones like cortisol and adrenaline get out of whack, and the pros and cons of taking testosterone. We're rounding out this chapter by debunking one of the most harmful cultural myths about age and the desperate desire and countless cultural pressures we face, to look, feel, and stay forever young.

Let this chapter inform, educate, and empower you to better understand what may be happening hormonally.

THE ENERGY DRAINS

Energy Drain #1:
Your Adrenals Have Screwed Up Cortisol Production

Your adrenals are tiny little glands that sit above your kidneys. They produce hormones that help regulate your blood sugar levels, immune system response, metabolism, digestion, and more.

Two hormones your adrenals create have a starring role in our exhaustion story: cortisol and adrenaline.

Let's look at cortisol first. *Cortisol* has a role in many processes of your body. It helps reduce inflammation. It helps control your metabolism, and it helps regulate your blood sugar levels by releasing glycogen (glucose) reserves from the liver and muscles.

Say you're going about your day and your body needs glucose, i.e., energy. There's nothing readily available, and maybe you're hitting the slopes and don't have time for a snack. Your body's not using its fat reserves either because (a) it's not a fat-burning machine or (b) the fat's busy holding mercury so you don't poison yourself.

If your body doesn't have the glucose it needs, it calls up your adrenals and says, "Hey, make some cortisol, so we can get that glycogen." Then your adrenals get to work making some cortisol, which gets released into your bloodstream. That cortisol helps to release your glycogen reserves.

This process also happens at night when you're sleeping and your brain needs energy to do all its healing and restorative work. Your adrenals get cranking. They make some cortisol, which releases your glycogen reserves. Your brain gets fed and it's happy.

Cortisol also has another role, and that's responding to stress. Cortisol is actually known as the stress hormone. It boosts energy and helps to motivate you to manage your daily stressors. We're coming back to cortisol in a second, so hang tight. We have to introduce another player in our cast of characters.

When you're stressed, your adrenals will create and release both cortisol *and* adrenaline.

Adrenaline is a hormone crucial to regulating your fight-or-flight response. It's the stuff you use if you're out on a long hike, turn a corner, and find yourself face-to-face with a bear. Adrenaline jacks up your system to get you in and out of an emergency quickly.

Adrenaline can also get used at night if you don't have enough glycogen reserves to feed your brain. Maybe your blood sugar levels are too low. If that's the case, your adrenals will bust out some adrenaline. They've got to wake you the hell up so you can grab a midnight snack and get those blood sugar levels higher.

What we just described is very natural and normal. Here's where our story goes off the rails. Cortisol is meant to be used during the day. But for short bursts. Adrenaline is meant to be used in emergencies only. For some people, their adrenals are pumping cortisol and adrenaline into their bodies far too often.

The reasons for this vary. Blood sugar issues can cause it, and so can stress. We've pounded the drum of our broken world throughout the book. Many of us lead stress-filled lives. We're stuck in fight-or-flight mode all day. That means our bodies are making cortisol and adrenaline from the moment we wake to when sleep finally comes, and it's taking a toll on our adrenals. "The adrenal glands are triggered when we are under constant, ongoing stress," said Dr. Meghan Walker, a naturopathic doctor who specializes in optimizing the health and performance of entrepreneurs. "Your adrenals can't see out, so they can't differentiate whether we are on a pilgrimage with our tribe and we are lacking water, or whether we have a really hard deadline in another 10 days."[1]

Our adrenals have become 24/7 cortisol-manufacturing plants. This is bad news.

You start piling up the years, and eventually your adrenals could crash. They may hit a point where they're like, "Dude, I'm out. I'm done. I can't keep up this pace any longer." When this happens, the first thing to go are your cortisol levels. They drop, and now you don't have the juice to get through your day, and you get hammered by fatigue.

Energy Drain #2: Your Cortisol Patterns Have Flipped

Cortisol also plays a major role in helping to regulate your sleep/wake cycles. When you wake up, it's cortisol that helps you get out of bed.

You open your eyes, and your brain gets a little stressed thinking about the day to come. That's not a bad thing. That little burst of stress signals to your adrenals to get some cortisol so it gets going.

In a natural world, your cortisol would spike in the morning. As the day wears on, it should fall as your melatonin (which helps put you to sleep) starts to rise.

But that wave isn't happening.

"I see a lot of people who are exhausted who also have a flipped cortisol pattern," explained Dr. Heidi Hanna. "Unfortunately, with most people who are chronically tired, whether it's psychological or physical, are showing this reversed pattern. There really is something going on at a systemic level. This isn't just that they're weak or that they should be pushing through it (the exhaustion)."[2]

If you have flipped cortisol patterns, then your cortisol levels will be low in the morning, and you won't have the energy or motivation to function. Then as the day passes, your levels will start to rise, spiking before you go to sleep. Now you can't rest and recover, because cortisol is flooding your body and you're ready to go.

There are many theories as to why these flipped cortisol patterns are showing up. One being we just can't turn off our brains. We're on overdrive with our thoughts and the stress from our modern world.

We're also overstimulated with scary news headlines that keep our adrenaline pumping. We go to sleep looking at news headlines on our devices, and wake up looking at news headlines on our devices—all emitting that dangerous blue light that lets our cortisol spike, keeps our melatonin low, and disrupts our pineal glands.

Many people are also caught in horrible work cultures. They've got unrealistic bosses who place unreasonable deadlines and expectations on them. They're caught living in deadline city, trying desperately to keep up with unrelenting workloads that have them sacrificing their sleep. If you're tired and really want to sleep, but you aren't allowing yourself that rest, then your brain is forced to call up your adrenals saying, "Hey, this person wants to keep going, we're not done marching, make it happen." Cue your adrenals pumping out cortisol to keep you up.

To return to your natural cortisol pattern, you have to manage your stress, reset your circadian rhythm by going to bed at normal hours, and reduce your blue light exposure at night. All of this sounds like work, but it's the opposite—it implies chilling the hell out more often and not feeling guilty about looking like a bum for a while. It means becoming okay with the idea that your recovery may involve doing a bit less now so you can heal.

Energy Drain #3:
You're Pilfering Cortisol from Other Hormones

Your brain is like an overlord that's willing to sacrifice every organ in your body to keep itself alive. If it needs cortisol to get its sugar supply rolling, to manage stress, or to deal with inflammation, it's going to get it, no matter the cost.

Even if your adrenals respond with "Hey, we're out of cortisol because this person's been running us pretty ragged for 20 years," it doesn't matter. Your brain doesn't care. It wants its cortisol, and it will have its cortisol. If your adrenals are functioning normally, no big deal.

If they aren't, that's a problem.

Your adrenals become forced to scramble to make more cortisol. What they do is start stealing the raw materials for cortisol from other hormones they're supposed to make. It's like they've clear-cut a forest, but they still need the timber for their ships, so they move on to another.

Your adrenals make a variety of hormones, including sex hormones that control the growth of reproductive organs (testicles and ovaries). One hormone your adrenals may tap is pregnenolone. This is starter material for other sex hormones, including testosterone, progesterone, and estrogen.

When your body starts tapping into pregnenolone for cortisol, you can develop what's called *pregnenolone steal*. Now your sex hormones malfunction, and your sex organs along with it. If you're a guy, maybe you stop getting erections. If you're a woman, you may skip your periods or struggle with fertility issues.

It's like playing dominos. One hormone falls and others follow. When your testosterone levels are low, you may lose lean muscle mass (and mitochondria with it). Body fat could also increase, and your skin may become drier.

It's not just testosterone your adrenals pilfer from. They hit up progesterone, which is a calming hormone. When you have low progesterone, you feel more irritable and may even have trouble sleeping. Your adrenals may also steal from estrogen too. When these levels drop, women may get hot flashes (like they would during menopause), irregular periods, and they may feel depressed. Estrogen is believed to be linked to serotonin, a neurotransmitter in the brain that boosts happiness.

This is just a sampling of the many and varied side effects that can arise when you've got your adrenals siphoning cortisol from other hormones. And all roads lead back to you becoming exhausted.

Energy Drain #4:
You're Using Testosterone as a Long-Term Solution

Taking testosterone has become one of the go-to treatments. If you go and tell your doctor you're tired, your testosterone levels will be one of the first they test.

If they see it's low, they may say, "Oh, I know why you're tired! Here, take this hormone replacement and you'll feel better." Admittedly, you will feel better. If you can barely move and your testosterone levels have flatlined, then you take some, you're going to stand upright. Testosterone helps "juice" more energy out of your cells and tells the body that growth is happening, so let's move this animal!

Another reason you feel better is because testosterone is helping your body make more lean muscle. Remember, the leaner muscle, the more powerhouse mitochondria get bigger and stronger. Now your energy producers are humming. That's why you feel better.

Testosterone also helps enhance moods, increasing competitiveness and mental sharpness. People with low "T" oftentimes feel defeated and depressed, so when their "T" increases, they feel more accomplished, satisfied with their lives, and ready to conquer the world. Testosterone can really give them an edge.

But there can be some dark sides to relying on testosterone—or any hormone. If you start taking hormones like testosterone, it signals to your body to stop making them. Why waste energy producing hormones it doesn't need? This isn't good. You want your body to naturally produce testosterone and other hormones on its own. The longer your body's dependent on an outside hormone supply, the harder it is to get your body pumping them out again.

Another downside is that sometimes when men start taking testosterone, it may get transferred to making dihydrotestosterone, which is a sex hormone and steroid. You'll have more energy for sure, but if your dihydrotestosterone is too high, you could lose your hair and be at a higher risk for prostate cancer.

Some people may also aromatize testosterone to estrogen. This is a chemical conversion that transforms a molecule by pulling off a hydrogen atom. Now your testosterone is being stripped down and made into estrogen. Think guys who have "man boobs." This may already have happened before the testosterone supplements came into play. If you're a dude and you're struggling with weight and you have "man boobs," testosterone won't help you—it's going to make your estrogen issues worse. It'll make you lose hair faster and increase your cancer risk. For women, if you're already tired and choking on estrogen, this downward spiral makes it worse.

Finally, if you look closely at the health profile of someone taking testosterone, you will likely find their cortisol levels are screwed up. They often have metabolic disorders and other endocrine issues too.

Energy Drain #5:
You're Encouraged to Stay Forever Young

We can't leave the subject of hormones without calling attention to one of the major pressures facing everyone today: the pressure to stay young.

Our media and culture seem to create an atmosphere of fear and shame around aging, and sometimes it's this desire to keep ourselves looking young that leads us to taking hormone replacements. We have antiaging creams and other products marketed to us regularly, and we're encouraged to stay wrinkle-free and to hide any gray and white hair. These are pressures that men and women face on the daily.

Wanting to feel young, to have your body feel vibrant and strong and filled with life is one thing. Yet it's different from being told by the media that you need to stay young. We live in a bullshit culture that's telling us to drink from some mythical fountain of youth that doesn't exist, nor should it.

That notion is damaging. It's toxic. And it's draining vital life force and energy from people.

Your body will change as you age, and during some of that transition, you may feel less energetic.

Personal Quest (Pedram)

I used to think I was a superhero. I had planned everything in my life perfectly. I was running a successful business, writing books, hosting podcasts, and making documentaries.

My wife and I also had our first baby on the way. We had a due date, so I had planned my life all the way up to when the little guy was supposed to arrive.

"Man plans, and God laughs," as the saying goes. The baby showed up *two weeks early*—that was definitely not part of our plan or schedule. It felt like I had been standing on a beach, watching a beautiful sunset, and then I was swept into the sea by some monster wave that rose up out of nowhere and crashed into me. For the next two years, it felt like I was swimming as a hard as I could just to get my head above the water, just so I could take another breath before the next wave crashed over me, pulling me under again.

Suddenly this thing that I had taken for granted called "sleep" was stolen from me. I didn't drink coffee until my son was born. For the first time, I struggled to exercise; I didn't feel like it. I didn't even feel like having sex.

I was underwater with way more commitments than I had the energy and time to handle, but it felt like I didn't have a choice. I had to muscle through no matter how exhausted I had become. For two years, I pulled from my adrenals running off cortisol and then snagging more from other hormones until there was nothing left. I became stressed out, wired and tired, and exhausted.

It was a huge reconciliation for me. I was a meditation guy, a kung fu guy, and this leader in the health and wellness environment, and I was sucking fumes. There was no way I could sustain my pace—and it was going to leave my wife a widow and my son fatherless.

So, for one winter solstice, I gave myself permission to pare back my professional obligations, allow myself to focus on my family, learn to better manage my stress, start new daily practices, and rest more so my adrenals and hormones could heal.

For the next couple of months, I went inward. I allowed myself to sleep when I needed to. I journaled. I went on long walks in nature and practiced more qigong. I started setting better boundaries around working, saying no to more projects and yes to the ones that brought in the money and allowed me to support my family, grow my business, and help more people heal. I cut back on caffeine and used adaptogens to help support my adrenals and hormones—just like I had counseled so many of my patients to use. I let go of self-judgments too, telling myself it was okay to be tired and to take it easy until I regained my energy. I spent more time with my wife, helping her with the nightly and daily feedings, diaper changes, laundry, dishes, and the daily tasks that raising a toddler brings. I focused on bringing more balance into my daily life.

It took about six months for my adrenals and hormones to recover, my body to heal, and my energy to rebound, but it worked.

That was about five years ago, and I haven't had an issue since.

TESTS

If you head to a doctor to test your adrenals, many will check certain hormone levels. Low levels are thought to be a sign of adrenal issues. What hormones will many practitioners want to look at? Here are some of the top ones you can expect.

Cortisol

Checking cortisol levels at different times in the day is a way for doctors to see if you're suffering from flipped cortisol patterns. They can check your cortisol levels by testing urine, saliva, or blood.

ACTH hormone test

This is thought to be the most specific test for diagnosing adrenal issues. Your doctor will measure cortisol levels in your blood before and after they give you an injection of a synthetic form of ACTH.[3]

Blood tests

A comprehensive blood test can measure hormone levels and show imbalances. Your doctor may test hormone levels, including estrogen, progesterone, testosterone/DHEA, and cortisol. They may also test the SHBG (sex hormone binding globulin) levels in your blood. SHBG is a protein that carries hormones such as testosterone, estradiol (an estrogen), and dihdrotestosterone (DHT) throughout the body.

DHEAS tests

Measuring DHEAS levels can help a doctor determine how your adrenals function. DHEAS are typically ordered with other tests. For men, the tests measure testosterone and several male hormones. For women, they may be ordered with hormone tests, including estrogen, testosterone, prolactin, and more.

Saliva Test

Your doctor can measure some hormone levels through a saliva test. These hormones include testosterone, estradiol, and progesterone.

THE ENERGY REMEDIES

Energy Remedy #1:
Make Adaptogens Part of Your Diet

If your adrenals are shot, what can you do? In the short-term, you may be able to use what are called *adaptogens*. These are natural remedies that can help support your body to adapt to stressors in your life. Many indigenous people living all over the world, often in harsh climates, use these herbs to help their bodies to adapt. It can boost systems when they're running low, or calm overexcited, overstimulated systems. For example, in Siberia, people make a soup out of *Eleutherococcus*, which is similar to ginseng, that they eat all winter long when it's 20 degrees below zero.

In Chinese medicine, the adaptogen *Astragalus membranaceus* is used, which is put into soup and given to kids during the winter months to strengthen their immune system. It's also anti-inflammatory.

When people are chronically exhausted, many functional medical practitioners turn to adaptogens. They're perfect for our modern, often stressed-out, world. And they're perfect to help support the adrenals and your stress levels.

You can take them at night and drink them as a tea or tonic. With adaptogens, you can take them as long as you need.

A word of caution. Most physicians suggested you should test your cortisol levels first. Adaptogens can increase or decrease cortisol levels, so you'll want to know where you're starting so you select the right herb.

Here are some of the best adaptogens for your adrenals:

Ashwagandha. This is used for people who have either high or low cortisol, and are extremely exhausted. It's also fantastic for sleep. It can give you the energy you need when you need it, and dials your energy back when you should be resting and recovering.

People who are "wired and tired" when their bodies are exhausted but who can't get their brains to turn off usually do well with this.

Rhodiola. Rhodiola gives you energy. It can also ramp it down. It's a gentle herb that is great for helping people rebuild their systems if exhaustion has knocked them down.

Holy Basil. This herb is great at calming and soothing your system. It will also uplift you.

Eleutherococcus. Also known as Siberian ginseng, it's popular with people who are struggling with chronic, long-term stress. It will bring your energy up or down, depending on what you need.

Ginseng and/or Licorice. These are useful if your cortisol levels are on life-support. Both bring up cortisol levels, and can help them to stay up. If you have high blood pressure or high cortisol levels, then skip both.

Lemon Balm. This can help you sleep at night, and is amazing for anxiety and overall anxiousness—all issues that can arise when you're exhausted.

Maca. Maca is known for its ability to balance hormones. Unlike other adaptogens, maca is a radish, which Peruvians eat often.

B Vitamins. B vitamins help nourish the adrenals and help with your stress response and mood. Taking a B-complex vitamin in the morning can help to boost your energy.

Energy Remedy #2: Slow the Hell Down

Your adrenals and hormones, especially flipped cortisol patterns and issues with low cortisol, have a lot to do with how you're interpreting stress. It has to do with exposing your body to harmful stress that keeps it in fight-or-flight mode. Part of the equation here is learning to slow down and to be gentle with yourself.

We know it may sound a little cheesy for us to say, "Be gentle with yourself." Yet we're going to say it, and we're going to keep saying it. Both of us need that message just as much as everyone else. That permission is missing culturally, and it's driving us into the ground. There's a permission missing in our lives to slow down, to honor our bodies, and to give them what they need.

Every time you feel tired, instead of saying, "I'm going to honor my beautiful body by taking a break and letting my energy levels reset," you probably tell yourself, "Okay, you stupid loser, why don't you be more like Cindy over there, go drink some coffee, get a face lift, and you'll be fine? Suck it up."

That mindset is destroying you. When you don't rest, when you're overworked, and you're pushing and pushing yourself, then you're pushing and pushing your adrenals and hormones to the point of failure.

Then you wind up exhausted and flat on your back.

Pedram has done a lot of backcountry backpacking. Early on, he'd stack his pack full, and on day one, he'd keep too fast of a pace and find himself panting by the side of the trail—only to watch the older and more experienced hikers breeze by him as if they were strolling through a damn meadow.

He learned over time to maintain a cadence that helped him stay "under his breath." This means always slowing down and being able to talk without losing his breath. As he developed this, he started to use this metaphor across his life. Where else was he getting ahead of himself? How could he slow down and stay under his breath?

Slow and steady truly wins the race—it's not just some silly kids' fable about a tortoise and a hare. Be the tortoise and live longer. Slow down and build a healthy fire in your belly.

There's a place for grit and determination and pushing through. We could teach a master class on that. But you also need to give yourself the space to feel safe, comfortable, cared for, and peaceful.

A lot of us don't have that at any point in our days. We live in a very masculine culture that has all but snuffed out the feminine. But life is duality. Nature is duality. The masculine and feminine both exist for a reason, and each of us—regardless of our gender—needs to learn how to tap into both sides.

This is our plea to you. If you can't grant yourself permission to rest and relax and slow down, let us. Let us say: Give your body what it needs, what it wants. It's okay to let yourself rest and recharge, that's a part of slowing down. Give your body a chance to stop cranking on your adrenals to push cortisol or adrenaline through the system.

"We don't prioritize the recharge nearly as much as we do the spending, the giving, the going, the rushing, the hurrying," said Dr. Heidi Hanna. "We can heal and we can have more sustainable energy, where we still have those great ups, those peak performance moments, but the only way we can do that is to also come back down, calm down, and recharge."[4]

Talk a long walk outside. Go for a hike in the woods. Meditate. Take a yoga class. Have sex. Go to the beach or a lake. Get in the water and swim. Soak in a tub. Play with your kids—let them remind you how fun life can be.

Just do activities that calm the fight-or-flight mode. When you do this, you help bring balance back to your adrenals and hormones, and you'll feel better. Remember to get restful and restorative sleep. Many of the lifestyle changes we talked about earlier can help you with your adrenals and flipped cortisol patterns.

Energy Remedy #3: Double-Check That Gut

Everything in your body is interconnected. It should come as no surprise that your gut plays a crucial role in keeping your hormones balanced. Your gut has specific bacteria that help metabolize your hormones. We covered this in Chapter 3: The Gut and Immune System, so here's our plug to reread that chapter and check out the remedies.

Particularly, mind your prebiotic and probiotic foods.

Prebiotics contain loads of fiber, which your friendly bacteria love. Remember, adding raw garlic, raw or cooked onions, asparagus, oats, leeks, flaxseed, apples, and bananas can help bolster the friendly gut bacteria.

Probiotics can include foods like kimchee, yogurt, sauerkraut, dill pickles, miso, and tempeh.

Energy Remedy #4: Get to the Root

"It takes more than hormones to fix your hormones," said Dr. Anna Cabeca, an ob-gyn and women's health expert. "You have to incorporate practices and lifestyle habits, nutrient habits, and supplements that will help you, but that depends what each individual is dealing with."[5]

Dr. Cabeca echoed what we heard from many hormone specialists. Just taking testosterone likely won't solve your exhaustion problems forever. You have to dig deeper to understand *why* your levels are so low to begin with. This is true for any hormone level that's out of balance.

A good physician may use testosterone or other hormones to jumpstart your body, but a great physician will use these as a quick fix, while working with you to understand the root cause.

If your doctor wants to put you on testosterone, please don't just take it. Find out the plan for the next few months, and then the next two years.

In fact, don't let *any* medical professional hand you a prescription or treatment plan without talking to you about the long-term strategy. If we've just described your doctor, drop them, and don't look back. Find a better doctor who will work with you on addressing the underlying issues.

The root causes for adrenal and hormone issues are varied. It could be that your stress levels are too high and you need to better manage them throughout the day. Maybe it's your diet, like if you're eating too many processed foods.

Maybe your toxin exposure is too high. "A tremendous amount of chemicals are endocrine disruptors, which means they start replacing estrogen, progesterone, thyroid hormones, and others," explained Dr. Darin Ingels, a naturopathic physician who specializes in environmental medicine, Lyme disease, and autism.[6] Endocrine disruptors interfere with your body's ability to naturally produce hormones, because the chemicals mimic the hormones, tricking your body into believing it's producing what it needs. If you happen to use personal care products, creams, lotions, perfumes, or anything with a color or fragrance made with phthalates, then your hormones may be affected, causing your exhaustion. Phthalates are known to be endocrine disruptors.

Will getting to the root of your adrenal and hormonal imbalance take a little more work? Probably.

Is it worth it? Absolutely.

Energy Remedy #5: Embrace Your Life Stage

The only way out of the media hellscape that encourages you to stay forever young is to start shifting your mindset around aging. We're not saying this is easy. But if you want to regain control over your energy, you have to stop letting the culture drain it away.

Instead of pretending aging doesn't happen, what if you embraced your life at each stage? What if you celebrated where you were, no matter what? There is such a beauty to understanding our mortality, a beauty to moving through each season and transformation of our lives, and milking it for all that it's worth.

You're not going to feel as youthful at 60 as you did at 20. You're not going to feel like staying out all night dancing. Hell, we're in our forties; we don't want to dance all night. We do that, we're done for a month. And that's fine. We're dads to young kiddos.

The more you push against the natural rhythms of life and nature, of which you're a part, the more it vamps your energy. Don't let it. Break free from our broken world and culture that tells and shows you that youth and staying young are all that matter.

Embrace whatever stage of life you're at. Stop comparing yourself to other people, especially the people you see plastered on your screens and in the magazines. Try tuning in to your body and ask what it wants, whether it's a gentle stroll outside or a bowl of soup. Maybe it's curling up in bed with a cup of hot tea and a good novel. Or maybe it's pouring a glass of wine (not the bottle) and calling your college roommate to catch up. Meet your energy levels where they are. Work with the rhythms of your body, with the rhythms of the seasons.

We're willing to bet you'll discover new energy and vitality the moment you stop trying to swim upstream and fighting against the natural order of the world.

Embrace all of you, for who and where you are in each moment of your life. Every stage, every age, is beautiful. You just have to see it.

Energy Remedy Bonus: Cultivate Smile Wrinkles

Wrinkles—a sure sign of aging or something else? Our culture does a lot to get rid of them. Can we say, Botox?

Here's a revolutionary idea. Maybe it's time to just let go.

Seriously, let's put down the needles and embrace our wrinkles. Let's try to make more of them. One of the most beautiful, most striking images in the world is seeing an older person whose eyes twinkle and who has smile wrinkles around their eyes and mouths.

These people overflow with the abundance of the universe. Power, and wisdom, and joy radiate from them. It's like they're fully operational power plants glowing from the inside out.

It comes from actually loving life—*your life*—and yourself. A really easy, costs-no-money, and takes-no-time way to get these wrinkles is to just start smiling more.

Even if you don't feel like it. Smile. Smile when you work. Smile at strangers you see in the grocery store. Smile at the driver next to you while you both sit at the red light. Smile while you're on the phone or typing an email.

Just smile.

And let your wrinkles reflect something deeper and more profound than just "getting old." Let them reflect a life well-lived, filled with laughter and joy.

SOLUTION

Before trying IVF, Bethany decided to see a functional medicine doctor. It turned out her adrenal health and hormone levels were intimately tied to her desire to procreate. Biological systems need energy to pass life from one generation to the next, so she had to get her adrenal health and hormones working optimally again.

Bethany's doctor recommended lifestyle and behavior changes and told her, "Don't even think about getting pregnant right now. I need six months to get you healthy."

Bethany heeded her doctor's advice and began focusing on how she could get healthier.

Six months later, Bethany had adopted a daily meditation practice. She went to yoga a few times a week, started walking outdoors for 30 minutes a day, cut down on her caffeine intake, and used various adaptogens to help nourish her adrenals. She also removed gluten and dairy from her diet, which had caused some food intolerances and polycystic ovary syndrome (a condition that creates hormonal imbalances and can make conceiving difficult). Bethany also practiced letting go of the need to get pregnant, which we want to honor is incredibly difficult to do. She focused more on living every day, practicing healthy habits and behaviors, nourishing her mind, body, and soul, spending quality time with her husband, talking to her sister more regularly, and giving herself permission to just be.

With these lifestyle and dietary changes and letting go of the need to get pregnant, Bethany slowly began her road to recovery. Eight months later, she conceived, and today Bethany is happily the mother of two children.

PERSONAL CHALLENGE

For one week, add one "be gentle with yourself" practice into your daily life. It doesn't matter what. It just has to be something that relaxes you, that makes you feel like you're taking care of yourself and your body, and that helps you to slow down. It doesn't have to be for a long period of time, although we won't stop you if you're adding an hour of self-care a day to your life.

If you have to, start small. Give yourself permission to have at least 10–15 minutes just for you. At first, it may be tough to slow down, but after a week, we bet you're going to want to up those minutes.

CHAPTER 8

The Brain

Frank had earned his M.B.A. and then became a top research analyst for one of the largest investment banks on Wall Street. For the first few years, Frank was on top of his game and was seen as an up and coming star.

His job was to look at macro trends in the economy. He spent hours every day pouring over charts and spreadsheets and making recommendations to his fund on whether an investment was a good deal or not.

It was a very high-pressure job with millions of dollars on the line. He was only as good as his last recommendation. If he picked a loser and his bank bet people's pension money on a recommendation that went wrong, then the guillotine would fall quickly. This meant Frank was incredibly stressed out trying to make sure his recommendations and analysis were *perfect*.

Frank had a lot on the line, not to mention he was paid extremely well for his brainpower—power that was starting to flicker. Year after year he was losing focus. The amount of data that kept coming in was immense, and he was always on a deadline. He was okay crunching the numbers, but each in-depth analysis and report was getting a little harder to put together and taking longer too.

He used to be able to work 8 hours without a break, and sometimes he could log 12- to 14-hour days too with no problem. Now he can barely concentrate more than 2 hours. He's falling behind with his workload, and he's having to put in regular 12-hour days just to keep up. He's rarely sleeping. He's either staying up late trying to get through his pile, or he's lying in bed stressed about his work quality and his never-ending responsibilities.

He's beat—physically, mentally, and emotionally—and desperate for a solution that will bring back his brainpower and energy. Frank went to a local health food store and tried different supplements. None have worked. He thought maybe there was something really wrong with his brain, so he went for brain scans, but those didn't show any issues. He also went to a psychologist who told him he was stressed out (he already knew that).

Frank thinks that the problem may be with his career and that he needs to change it. But he doesn't really want to. He likes being the numbers guy and analyzing trends. Still, he may have no other choice because the work feels harder than ever, and his brain is fried.

THE PROBLEM

As we near the end of our exhaustion road trip, we have to warn you, this is the tough love chapter. We're going to challenge how you've been living your life and the decisions you've made that have led you to this book. Many of the remedies won't be quick or easy, but they could make some of the biggest differences in your life.

At times, it may seem like we're repeating ourselves, like we double back on previous chapters and recommendations for healing. This is on purpose. Everything about exhaustion is interconnected, and all roads lead to your brain.

Your brain is like a lightbulb. When it's turned on, you feel like you have energy, like you have the ability to think clearly, and to make good rational decisions. You also feel excited, engaged, and happy about life.

When you're exhausted, you don't feel any of this. You feel like you're living 24/7 with a Sunday-morning hangover, and wondering if your brain even works right.

We call this *brain fog*. The term covers a lot of ground. You may feel less sharp, foggy, cloudy. You may feel like you can't reason, think through, or problem solve very well. You may feel confused, or like your mind just goes blank, where it's just slow to process. You may struggle to remember events, people, or words. You may also feel anxious, worried, lethargic, or depressed. Brain fog may trample your mood, and you may lack the motivation for life.

So many people are living with brain fog, and some don't even know it. It takes a level of self-awareness to realize our minds aren't operating at their highest capacity. It's really tough to know when you're off, which can quickly spiral into a vicious cycle. You can't always recognize the patterns of behavior that have led you to this moment because the organ being affected is the same one that's supposed to be doing your thinking and helping you recognize the bad behaviors and poor choices. The very thing you're perceiving the world through, the maker of your reality, is compromised.

Brain fog can be tricky to reverse too. Unlike our other chapters, brain fog is not a cause for your exhaustion. It's a symptom, often the most obvious one. If your gut bacteria are off, if you're not getting restorative sleep, if you're eating a diet too rich in sugars and carbs, if you're not getting enough exercise, or if you're exposed to too many toxins, your brain will be affected. Your light will be dimmed. It will flicker and you will feel like crap.

To fix brain fog, you have to find and treat the underlying cause for it. In this chapter, we're going to help you identify some potential reasons for it, including energy and nutrient deficiencies, inflammation, chronic stress, trauma, and lifestyle choices.

Our intention is to inspire and empower you to keep seeking the truth. If the truth eventually leads you back to addressing some of the previous energy drains, then so be it. Follow whatever path you need to take.

When you fix the underlying issues, you will fix your brain. When you fix your brain, your lightbulb gets brighter. When your lightbulb gets brighter, your mind becomes clearer and sharper, and you feel lighter, happier, and more excited. Then you will have the energy and motivation you need to live the big life that we know you yearn for.

Be strong in this chapter. Be focused, be determined, be resilient. Your brain is extraordinary, and when you get that firing, you live an extraordinary life.

THE ENERGY DRAINS

Energy Drain #1: Your Brain Needs More Energy

Your diet, gut, and brain are interconnected. We've mentioned this before, but your brain needs a lot of juice to work. While it represents about 2 to 5 percent of your total body weight, it consumes a whopping 20 percent of your energy.[1]

For many people battling exhaustion and brain fog, it's because their brain is simply not getting the energy it needs to function right. There can be many reasons for this, so let's break down some of the major ones.

Imbalanced Gut Bacteria

If your gut bacteria are off, then you won't digest your food correctly. If you're not digesting your food, your brain isn't getting the glucose (sugar) it needs to function right and you're left in a fog. (You're also left with uncomfortable GI issues like constipation, being super gassy, loose stools, and other bodily functions that we pretend never happen to us.)

We're also learning that an imbalanced gut can affect the vagus nerve. The vagus nerve is the tenth cranial nerve that runs from the brain to various organs including those that make up your digestive tract. It's the most elaborate nerve and, believe it or not, there's actually a two-way communication happening when you eat.

Your brain sends a message down the vagus nerve to your digestive organs saying, "Hey, get ready and go ahead and digest that food."

What we're learning is that the bacteria in the gut impact the nerves all the way up this channel. If you have an overabundance of bad bacteria in your gut, they can start climbing out and up along various nodes of the vagus nerve, eventually traveling all the way to your brain. Researchers are now tracing Parkinson's and Alzheimer's to these bacteria and learning that they can spend *fifteen years* making their way up the vagus nerve from the gut to the brain.

Not only can the bad bacteria affect your long-term health, it also can give you brain fog while slowly shutting down your system.

Too Many Sugars and Carbohydrates

Studies are finding that your brain does better when it's powered by healthy fat instead of sugars and carbohydrates. If you needed one more reason to start shifting from carbs and sugars, this is it.

Too many people are still carb and sugar loading, and it's damaging their brainpower, not to mention it can lead to blood sugar issues, which can harm the brain. When your blood sugar spikes and drops throughout the day and night, your cognition and emotions go along for the ride too. You're left without the ability to think clearly and rationally, while simultaneously becoming angry, irritable, short-tempered—also known as *hangry.*

Plus, when you're used to fueling your body with carbs and sugars, switching to fueling with fat can take some work and time. It usually means you have to build up your mitochondria by getting some lean muscle mass—again, something that many people need to work on.

Not Enough Electrolytes

Your brain has two types of cells. One is *glial cells*, which we're going to talk about in the next section, and the other is *neurons*. Neurons carry out brain functions like smelling, cognition, emotions, vision, and movement by sending and receiving chemical and electrical signals.

Electrolytes are minerals like sodium, chloride, phosphorus, magnesium, calcium, and potassium that your body needs so the electrical signals work correctly. Our entire nervous system functions because of variance in electrical gradients between nerves. These electrolytes help make this happen. To keep it simple, they pass electrons back and forth along the channels of nerves in a chain reaction (think of a crowd doing "the wave") along a nerve cell. Take that and multiply it times a billion, and you'll get the scale at which this all happens throughout the body and brain. For this to work right, your brain and body need the balanced presence of the right minerals or electrolytes in your diet.

When your electrolyte balance is off, the electrical conductivity goes haywire, and your neurons start shutting down. When your neurons shut down, your organs, muscles, and tissues begin slowing down, and you're left feeling worn out—among other side effects.

Water Intake

You need to drink water, clean and toxin-free. It's as simple as that, yet most of us are dehydrated. We're not getting enough, and when we don't get enough, our system isn't able to flush and clean itself as well. Water builds blood volume to move our nutrients to where they need to go and shuttle toxins out of the body. When we don't drink enough water, toxins build up in our bodies and brains, and our nutrients don't get to where they need to go to give us energy.

Energy Drain #2: Inflammation Has Invaded Your Brain

We've already talked about how inflammation is bad for your body, but it's bad for your brain too. And when your body is inflamed, your brain gets inflamed.

"The biggest clue that someone has fatigue related to brain inflammation is, when they use their brain, they completely wipe out," said Dr. Datis Kharrazian. "They can't read for more than a couple paragraphs, but they may be able to go for a workout, they can do physical things, but they can't do cognitive things. And that's one of the huge red flags that there's something wrong with the brain."[2] When your brain is inflamed, it can turn on your glial cells to fight infection and inflammation. Normally, your glial cells support your neurons. At night when you're sleeping, glial cells go around to your neurons, pruning and clipping the branches so they can send and receive information efficiently.

Glial cells also help to wash away any toxins that the brain picked up during the day. They get rid of protein plaques like amyloid plaque that can eventually lead to dementia, Alzheimer's, or Parkinson's.

Your glial cells are unsung heroes, performing critical roles in your health and vitality. But when these cells turn on to battle inflammation, they no longer handle cleanup. That means all of those toxins and plaques start building up, and you're left feeling foggier and more susceptible to serious diseases down the road.

As Dr. David Perlmutter explained to us, inflammation can also compromise the function of our energy producers, our mitochondria, which affects our brain function.

> When we increase inflammation by not getting enough restorative sleep, by eating the standard American diet, we create a situation that's threatening our very ability to use fuel that we consume as a source to power our mitochondria, which then powers our cells.
>
> When you realize the brain, representing 2 to 5 percent, depending on your body, of the total body weight is, at rest, consuming 25 percent of your energy, you realize it's a very energy-hungry part of your body. Those mitochondria are in need of being fueled properly. Anything that damages mitochondrial function is going to manifest as defective brain function.[3]

When your body and brain are inflamed, it also compromises your mitochondria as they switch from producing energy to defending your cells. There are five primary causes of inflammation: a poor diet, stress, toxins, microbes, and allergens. If you want to stop inflammation, eat clean, sleep well, relax, avoid toxins, and take care of your gut.

Energy Drain #3: You're Drowning in Chronic Stress

We live in very unusual times. Our ancestors had stress in their lives, for sure. But it was mostly acute. Think someone—or something—was chasing or trying to kill them. Usually the situation ended quickly. They either got away, or they wound up dead.

That's not the case today. Now it seems many of us are drowning in chronic stress. It's death by a thousand papercuts. In fact, Americans are actually some of the most stressed-out people in the world.[4]

We're supposed to be a land of opportunity where people from all over the globe come to make better, happier, more prosperous lives for themselves and their families. Yet we're stumbling through life strung out on stress, anxiety, worry, and fear.

Is this really how we want to live? Is this really the American dream we're chasing? Of course not. No one's out there raising both hands saying, "Yes, please sign me up for all of this stress."

It can feel like you don't have a choice, like the world has gone to shit, that it's broken, and there's nothing you can do about it. It's true, we do live in a broken world.

It's also true that you have way more control over this world and your stress than you realize.

Your brain is ground zero. The story of stress begins here, with how you understand, perceive, and then respond to the world around you. To understand stress, you have to understand what triggers it. Cue the *amygdala*, an almond-shaped mass of neurons that lies deep inside your brain. It is a part of your *limbic system*, which handles emotions, memories, and arousal.

Think of your amygdala as the control center passing judgment and making decisions on how your nervous system will respond to an event. It uses past experiences, your values, and beliefs to differentiate between what's a threat and what's no big deal. When the amygdala senses trouble, it means war has arrived on your shores. Instantly, it sends a "Danger! Danger!" message through a pathway called the *HPA Axis* (hypothalamic pituitary adrenal axis) to your adrenals telling them to release cortisol and adrenaline.

As we mentioned earlier, that cortisol and adrenaline flood your system and bam! You're now in fight, flight, or freeze. That means your body stops pumping blood to organs like your liver and digestive system, and instead diverts it to your arms and legs, so you're prepared to do battle, run like hell, or hide for your life.

When you're in this fight, flight, or freeze state, blood flow to the *prefrontal cortex* in your brain also stops functioning fully. The prefrontal cortex is where your critical, rationale, and moral thinking lies. It's what separates you from the monkeys. This is full-brain thinking. Your left and right brain are communicating, and you're having killer insights that lead to genius ideas and solutions.

When you're in the gear of fear or when you're in stress brain, all of this goes away. The blood is diverted to lower brain centers. The challenge you face is that your amygdala is being bombarded with experiences it judges as terrifying *all the time*. Now you're left living what should be your best years as a stressed-out, scared-shitless, tail-tucked-between-your-legs animal.

Your body is constantly placed in wartime, so your liver isn't detoxing as much as it normally would when you were in a relaxed, resting state. Your digestive system isn't functioning optimally. Your mitochondria aren't producing as much energy either—they've been switched on to defend your cells.

No wonder you're exhausted. No wonder you can't think straight.

Energy Drain #4: Trauma Is Stealing Your Vitality

There is something else that turns on our fight, flight, or freeze response and indirectly steals our energy: *trauma*.

Trauma and fatigue often go hand in hand.

Trauma is a broader category than many people think. Experts categorize trauma as "Big T" or "little t." "Big T" traumas include being a victim of sexual abuse, physical abuse, or domestic violence; being in a natural disaster, a war, a mass shooting, or an accident; losing a child or loved one; and experiencing a pandemic or other large societal event, as well as witnessing a "Big T" event.

"Little t" traumas include emotional abuse, developmental trauma (this occurs during childhood when we are still developing), verbal abuse, neglect, divorce, betrayal (such as being cheated on), rejection, being shamed, death or a loss of a loved one (including a pet), chronic stress and feeling overwhelmed, and being bullied or harassed.

Trauma includes traumatic brain injuries (TBIs) that you get from a physical accident and post-traumatic stress disorder (PTSD) symptoms.

Any deeply disturbing, emotional, physical, or psychological experience that goes beyond our body's ability to cope with stress can leave a trauma imprint in our brains and bodies. This is especially true if you've experienced childhood trauma before the age of 18.

We don't talk about this often, but even the micro events that can happen daily, once a month, or once a year can become traumatic. It's like if someone called your idea stupid during your weekly team meeting, and instead of thinking to yourself, *Whatever, they're an idiot,* or *they're having a bad day,* you're consumed by thoughts like *I can't believe they said that. Next time I'm going to punch them out, or I'm going to tell them off. I won't let them get away with it.* You're sitting and stewing, and caught in this trauma-drama.

When we're carrying unresolved traumas, they can get easily triggered. If you have an association with a certain smell, sound, image, or even a word that traumatized you in the past, then every time you pick up that scent, every time you hear that sound, see that image, or hear a specific word, that good 'ol amygdala gets triggered again, and you have a stress response. Your cortisol and adrenaline race through your system. Your body shifts into fight, flight, or freeze, and you're on high alert, ready for danger.

In the end, you lose energy because you're burning it hot and fast trying to deal with your trauma response.

We're bringing up trauma because so many people don't realize it's stealing their life force. If this is the root of your exhaustion, then the only way to fix this drain is to go deep inside and resolve the past.

Energy Drain #5:
You're So Broke, You Can't Even Pay Attention

If your brain doesn't have the energy to operate, it can't do anything. You lose focus, then you make terrible decisions like drinking when you should be sleeping, eating crap foods, not exercising, and not taking care of your body and energy the way you should.

These bad decisions can lead you to become exhausted. Your brain becomes dull, and you feel listless. Then you make even worse decisions as you spiral down. Then you start beating yourself up for making these choices, which leads you to make even worse decisions.

Deeper and deeper you go. Now you're just zapped on every level—physically, emotionally, mentally, and spiritually, and it feels like there is no hope, like there's nothing you can do. This is just an illusion. You have more power than you realize; it just doesn't feel like it.

Personal Quest (Nick)

I have a TBI that I didn't even know I had for the longest time. I just knew my brain felt like it was constantly "on," where I couldn't shut off my thoughts. I was overthinking and overstressing on everything in my life, and frankly, it was making me miserable and tired, when I really shouldn't have been. I was eating well. I was sleeping regularly. I had a career and family I loved. Yet it always felt like I was on edge, where I had to be on high alert for the next "shoe to drop."

When I went to see my doctor, she suggested we try neuro-feedback. We used a QEEG (Quantitative Electroencephalogram), which involves hooking up little sensors to my head to measure my brain waves and frequencies in real time. We went through different conversation topics as visual and auditory stimuli to observe how my brain responded.

When we first started monitoring my brain waves, I was spiking bright red with Beta for over an hour. Beta brain waves are great for concentration and work, but Beta in high frequencies for pro-longed periods can lead to anxiety and stress. Turned out, I was stuck in Beta.

My doctor had me wear a heart rate variability monitor to measure stress levels. It's a fantastic tool for teaching you what it feels like when you're stressed out versus when you're in a relaxed state. During a neurofeedback session, my doctor would see I was in Beta and would instruct me to move to the Alpha state (brain waves related to relaxation and mediation and peace).

I'd focus on deep breathing and meditation and slowly I'd watch as the numbers on my wearable went down.

I'd wear the HRV monitor throughout the day, and as soon as I started overstressing or overthinking, the device would alert me. Then I'd take a few minutes to practice my breathing and meditate, and my heart rate and brain waves would return to normal.

Within a month, I had started to gain more control over my stress levels. With neurofeedback, the HRV monitor, deep breathing techniques, and meditation, I began to rewire my brain. Today, I no longer burn energy on unnecessary or useless thoughts.

TESTS

When it comes to testing in your brain, a functional medicine doctor is likely to hit up some of the earlier tests we talked about. Toxins, food sensitivities, adrenal and hormone imbalances, nutrient deficiencies—these are all fair game tests that may lead to fixing your brain challenges.

Remember, brain fog isn't the root of your exhaustion; it's a symptom that goes along with it.

THE ENERGY REMEDIES

Energy Remedy #1: Get More Energy to Your Brain

If your brain fog is caused by lack of energy, your quest is to fix your diet and gut. These are the basic building blocks to a brain that's supercharged. If you're not giving your brain the right fuel it needs, it's never going to take off.

The list of ways to remedy this energy drain is very long, and we don't have space for that here. What we can give to you are a few quick hits on where to direct your focus. If any suggestions sound familiar . . . good. Everything is connected, remember?

From Sugar to Protein, Healthy Fat, and Complex Carbs
We're not telling you anything you haven't already heard with this tip. Cut out the sugar. Cut out the simple, "fast" carbs, and get thee on a healthy, whole-foods diet loaded with protein, healthy fats, and complex carbs.

Boost Electrolytes
There are some great natural ways to boost your electrolytes if your levels are too low. Here are some of our favorite general ways to get those numbers up.

Load up on colored vegetables and fruits. If you're looking to generally boost electrolytes, make sure you eat lots of leafy green vegetables and bring on the color. You want a varied, rich diet that includes different colored, whole foods. (We're not talking chips or sugary cereals.) At your next meal, try eating, at a minimum, two different colored foods per meal. For example, carrots and blueberries, or a sweet potato and broccoli. Bonus—it's a great way to boost your friendly gut bacteria. For more magnesium, eat your beans, greens, nuts, and seeds, and for potassium add avocados, brussels sprouts, kale, broccoli, kiwi, green beans, and strawberries to your diet.

Pass the salt. While most people try to avoid too much salt, it's an important mineral for your neurons. If your brain is sluggish and you are on a low-salt diet, try adding in a pinch of seaweed to your soups, stews, and smoothies. Kombu, wakame, and dulse can easily deliver sodium and trace minerals to help your brain. If you have high blood pressure, always consult your physician about dietary changes so they can track your blood pressure closely.

Take an Epsom salt bath. Soaking in a salt bath is actually a good way to absorb magnesium. We've mentioned magnesium a bunch already. It's such a badass mineral and does so much to keep your body and mind healthy and happy.

Drink More Water

Want an easy water hack? Drink a glass as soon as you wake up. It's a great way to flush your system and get you ready for the day. And no, sports drinks don't count for hydrating. In fact, mountain spring water with the minerals left in tends to be the best option.

Energy Remedy #2: Reduce Brain Inflammation

Inflammation is brutal. Unless you're gunning for the "good stuff" and purposely trying to get some inflammation to build lean muscle, you want to do everything you can to eliminate inflammation. The million-dollar question on everyone's mind: How?

"You really have to look at diet, nutrition, lifestyle, and see what the triggering factors are," said Dr. Datis Kharrazian. "You can use anti-inflammatory natural compounds and nutraceuticals (food or food products that help to treat the problem) to block inflammation. You can improve your diet so it's not as inflammatory, and make sure you get plenty of sleep. It's a whole lifestyle approach. Brain inflammation is definitely not going to be fixed by taking a simple supplement. It's a serious clinical approach."[5]

We've already mentioned a bunch of remedies that can help reduce possible brain inflammation throughout the book. We won't bore you with retreading a familiar path, so below is a rapid-fire checklist with the chapter reference for you:

- Make sure you're eating the right anti-inflammatory diet—you shouldn't nosh on foods like gluten, dairy, grains, soy, and sugar that your gut can't digest. (See Chapter 3: The Gut and Immune System.)

- You have to make sure your gut bacteria are balanced. (See Chapter 3: The Gut and Immune System.)

- You have to make sure you're exercising to build strong and healthy mitochondria. (See Chapter 4: Exercise and Movement.)

- You have to make sure you're getting enough restorative sleep at night so your brain can detox. (See Chapter 5: Sleep and Recovery.)

- You have to make sure you're not exposing your body to toxins unnecessarily. (See Chapter 6: Toxicity.)

- You have to make sure you're eating enough fiber to help eliminate waste and make sure your liver functions properly. (See Chapter 6: Toxicity.)

You have the power to reduce and control inflammation, but that means you have to look at your lifestyle choices and make some changes to see a difference.

Energy Remedy #3: Reduce Your Stress Load

When you're chronically stressed, reducing it is a must, but it's not always easy. For a lot of people, it's about chipping away and making a commitment to regaining your sanity.

There's no one way or right way to go about it. You have to take stock of your life and commit to finding solutions that work for you.

Will this take some effort? Yes. Will it take lots of practice? Yes. Will this be a lifetime commitment? Yes. Like so much in our exhausted journey, there is no quick fix to crawling out from under the chronic-stress fog. But you have to take control over your brain. Otherwise, it's going to hijack your energy, and ultimately your life.

To help get you started, we've included some simple ideas below. Aim to make some small adjustments, some little tweaks, to your life so you can begin to feel the flow of energy return.

Give Your Thoughts to Your Journal

Journaling is such a great way to get thoughts out of your mind and released to the Universe so you don't have to carry the burden. You can grab an actual journal and hold a real pen, or type away on your computer. No censoring. No thinking. Just freewrite whatever comes to mind, whatever you're mad or stressed about, whatever you're feeling.

This is just for you, and it's a safe place to release your thoughts and emotions. You don't have to be a writer to use this process. It doesn't have to be long either. You can journal for 10 minutes in the morning or at night. Set a timer for 10 minutes and just go.

Another twist on this remedy is the popular *gratitude journaling*. It's popular because it works. Just focusing on what you're truly grateful for helps to reduce your stress and brings you into the present moment.

Experiment with when you do it. Try writing down five things you're grateful for before you go to bed, and/or as soon as you wake up. "Before you get out of bed, think about all the things you're grateful for," suggested Dr. Leigh Erin Connealy, a leader in the functional medicine field. "That puts every cell in peace, which is what we're trying to all achieve every day. If we have peace, we can handle emotion, we can handle our hormones better, we can handle how we eat. How we digest and absorb nutrients and everything."[6]

Let Mother Nature Unwind Your Mind

When was the last time you spent time outdoors? We've mentioned being in nature often because it's so effective. Mother Nature heals us. She quiets our racing minds, reduces our stress, and renews our vitality. What's not to love?

One study found that people who spent 80 minutes in the morning and afternoon in the forest experienced reduced pulse rates, significantly increased scores for vigor, and decreased depression, fatigue, anxiety, and confusion.[7]

You don't have to spend two and a half hours a day outdoors to reap the benefits—if you can, more power to you. Just start with 15 or 20. If you can, walk in the morning, at lunch, after work, or after dinner.

Being outdoors is also one of the best activities you can do with your family. Consider carving out time on a weekend to go to a local, state, or federal park, or a nature center. If you're far from the woods, find a park close to you and hang out next to a tree.

When you're outdoors, focus on being present. We spend so much time in our heads, talking to ourselves, replaying that stressful meeting, or worrying about what may happen tomorrow. Instead of thinking, pay attention to the color of the leaves. Look at their shape.

Notice the world around you. This activates your right brain, so you become more creative and better at problem solving.

Being in nature reenergizes, lowers stress, and activates right brain thinking so you show up feeling better, having more energy, and with a brain that's supercharged. That sounds like a win-win to us.

Plan to Relax on the Hour Every Hour

A lot of people need to train themselves to relax and reduce their stress. An effective tool is to set a timer so, once every hour, you stop what you're doing and take a five-minute sanity break. If that's too much, stop for a minute or two. You've got a phone with a timer in it—put it to use!

Do whatever you want. Get up from your desk and stretch. Do some squats. Close your eyes and breathe deeply through your nose and into your belly. Meditate.

What matters is you're slowing down your system and reminding your body and mind what it feels like to relax no matter what's going on around you.

Add Some Damn Joy

It's not about how you reduce your stress, just that you do it. Pick something you want to do. It could be something you once loved doing, but haven't had time for since you got married, had kids, and had to juggle life.

If gardening relaxes you, do it. If it's spending time outdoors, do it. If it's going to yoga or meditation class, do it. If it's reading or watching a movie, do it. If it's cooking or baking, if it's taking a bath, if it's playing make-believe with the kids, if it's playing a board game with your spouse, do it.

Give yourself permission to take a break, to relax, to enjoy life, and let your mind unwind. You will feel rejuvenated.

Say "No" More

Are you overcommitting? It's okay if you are. Most of us run into this at some point in our lives. We say yes when we really want to and should say no when we don't. Whether you're prone to people-pleasing; trying to be helpful; overestimating the time, energy, and effort something would take; or used to putting everyone before yourself, this is about setting and standing by your boundaries. It's about learning that you can say no and the sky won't fall.

In fact, you'll have even more energy and attention to give to the people, tasks, and experiences that you do say yes to. And that's a good thing.

Learn to Breathe

Your breath has a powerful, almost magical effect on your energy. By controlling your breathing, you can control your energy. Specifically, you can control whether you're stuck in fight, flight, or freeze, or if you're in rest and digest.

Most people are shallow breathers. They breathe from their chests only, and from their mouths. But when you breath slowly through your nose and deep into your belly, you can shift your nervous system into a slower, more peaceful, more relaxed state. All it takes is a few minutes, and you can move yourself from stressed to chill.

Try this: Breathe in through your nose down to the deepest point in your body (about three fingers below your naval) to the count of four and hold it for four seconds, before breathing out through your nose for another four count. Do this exercise three times. Focus on breathing into your belly. Your belly should rise, not just your chest.

Here's another great practice: breathe in for a count of four, then breathe out for a count of six. This really slows your heart rate.

You can use these breathing tricks anytime you're feeling a stress response or before a potentially stressful experience. You can do deep breath work before a meal, before bedtime, or before going into that meeting with your boss or hopping on that team conference call. You can use it when you're in the car and stuck in gridlock or wedged between strangers on your next subway or metro ride.

When you're chronically stressed, learning how to breath can be one of the most powerful exercises. It costs you nothing, and it's something you can do anywhere, anytime.

Eliminate the Stress

For some people, reducing the chronic stress load is about eliminating it. We can't walk you through how to do that—that would take an entire book. But what we can do is hold up the mirror and help you see where your stress may be originating. Ultimately, you have to be the one to decide whether you need to change your reaction to the stress or if you need to eliminate it entirely.

Consider, what keeps you up at night?

- Is your financial house in order?
- Are you happy in your relationship with your spouse or partner?
- Are you content with your relationship with your friends, relatives, or parents?
- Are you pleased with how you act with your kids?
- Do you like your job?
- Do you like your boss?
- Do you like your co-workers?
- Do you like your office and the overall culture?

All of these issues can be huge drains on your brain. If any of these pieces of your life are the main source for your overactive mental game, then it may mean you have to make some big life adjustments to course correct. These can be tough, for sure, but in the long run, you'll feel a heaviness and burden lift from your mind (and rest of your body too).

Try a Heart Rate Variability Monitor

We get it. You're looking for hacks to fix your brain. These are largely tough to come by, but there is one tool that many people are having amazing results using. It's called a *heart rate variability monitor* (HRV), and it measures your stress levels.

You can get these as a wearable like a watch. In fact, many of the watches out there have apps that'll calculate this for you. When you're stressed out and your heart rate shoots up, the watch will buzz. It's a fantastic tool to bring greater awareness into your body, so you can catch yourself when you're jacked up and hitting the fight, flight, or freeze mode. People often pair this with breathing techniques as a way to consciously and intentionally lower your stress levels.

It's so effective that some doctors we spoke with said their patients have come off antianxiety medication because they've used these monitors with breathing techniques—it's that powerful. (This isn't our endorsement for you getting off antianxiety meds if you're on them. That's something you should only do in consultation with your doctor.) While we'd never guarantee the same outcome for you, it's definitely worth looking into if you're someone who overstresses, overthinks, and generally feels anxious a lot.

Energy Remedy #4: Seek Help for Your Trauma

Let's be real, we can't give you a formula for healing your trauma in a couple of quick remedies. That's not only impossible, it would be highly insulting to you. Trauma is a very complex, very real issue that deserves a more thorough and respectful response.

This is our public service announcement, and medical disclaimer: There are entire books written on trauma. This one brief section will not, nor can it, cure you. It's meant to help you better understand one *possible* area in your life that may be draining your energy.

If you're reading this chapter and suspect that trauma may be at the root of your exhaustion issues, please do not be discouraged. This book is largely about helping you to unwind your exhaustion knot. There are so many factors that can lead to feeling exhausted, being unable to think straight, and virtually incapable of operating at a high level. Much of this book is designed to help bring more conscious understanding of what may be your unique situation.

If you suspect trauma may be at the root of your exhaustion, that's a *victory*. That means you're one step closer to regaining your vitality and turning the tide back in your favor. It means you have a direction to walk in instead of spinning in circles, wondering what the hell is going on and how to move forward.

If there's something unresolved—wherever it stems from— please, seek professional help. Yoga, qigong, meditation, and other mindfulness tools have their place, but they're probably not going to be strong enough if your trauma is really heavy.

For most people, releasing their trauma means seeking help from medical professionals like a therapist. If that's you, it's okay. You've got to deal with this, so let's go. Work with a therapist. Unpack what's been bottled up in a safe environment, with a trained professional, and you will begin to regain your energy.

In the meantime, we're sharing three specific techniques that we've both used to help us unlock and release various traumas in our own lives. Again, these aren't replacements for seeking more professional help. Just a few highlights to get you out of the gate.

Take the ACE Quiz

Many people have no idea they're even traumatized. If you're wondering whether trauma is playing a role in your exhaustion, there are some great tests that can help you figure out how traumatized you may be. One test we have respect for is the *ACE Quiz*. It takes about five minutes to complete, is free, and it looks at different types of childhood traumas and abuses you may have been exposed to before turning 18.

Floatation Therapy

One powerful way to unlock trauma and let the brain molt is the use of a sensory deprivation tank. These water chambers that allow you to float in complete stillness, darkness, and silence were popular in the 1960s and 1970s and have come back recently. The water is at body temperature, and the tank deprives the body of sensory input so we can turn the focus of our awareness inside.

Without all the data coming in, the brain starts to trip out. Many report hallucinations. It gives you the space to shed layers and go inward. It can be deeply relaxing and rejuvenating for most people. Others face a rocky road and have their trauma come up.

If that's the case, make your next stop to a therapist so you can release what's come up, instead of letting it sink back inside.

Neurofeedback

We have five brain waves that are associated with different parts of our brain and relate to anxiety, impulsivity, cognitive inflexibility, emotions, thoughts, and behaviors. Neurofeedback is such a badass tool because it can show you, in real time, what brain wave frequency you're lighting up.

Our five brain waves include:

1. Delta, a sleep state.
2. Theta, a daydreaming, relaxed state.
3. Alpha, a meditative, relaxed state.
4. Beta, a concentration state connected with work.
5. Gamma, a very high, very fast frequency.

Most neurofeedback won't touch Gamma, but what it does pick up is Beta. Beta (especially High Beta) and your amygdala can be close friends. When you're in Beta, you're very focused. You may even be analyzing perceived threats, mentally trying to find your way out of a maze, or solving a puzzle.

There's nothing wrong with Beta, but we can overdo it. That's where chronic stress and trauma especially come into play.

When trauma has been triggered, it's often difficult to stop your mind from overthinking, from overstressing, or from reliving a traumatic experience. When your body is in fear, in fight, flight, or freeze, your brain doesn't know how to turn off. It's stuck in the High Beta frequency.

Alpha is the key. It is the clutch between the different gears. If you know how to activate Alpha, which is associated with meditation and a relaxed brain and body, then you can retrain your amygdala to stop sensing danger around every corner. It means you can stop getting triggered by your external environment.

Neurofeedback helps teach you to identify your brain waves and to start rewiring your brain using meditation and relaxation techniques.

Energy Remedy #5: Make Small Changes First

You want to feel better? You want to feel like you have the energy to face your day, to meet any and all challenges, to feel vibrant, alive, happy, and excited for life?

You need your brain for that.

To get that lightbulb shining, *you* have to feed it the right foods. *You* have to give it the right electrolytes. *You* have to put yourself to bed, go to sleep, and let your brain rest. *You* have to exercise and move your body. *You* have to relax and stop the stress response.

You. You. You have to be master of your universe and make the right decisions to get your energy back on track. You will not wake up one day and have that lightbulb magically turn on. That's not how life works, and it's not how your brain works.

Putting your health first is not a selfish act, so please ditch the guilt, ditch the fear, and ditch the worry. We know it's easier said than done sometimes, but please really hear us. By making your own wellness your top priority, you will finally have all the energy you dream of to be there for your family and your work. Everybody in your orbit wins.

The promised land of vitality and vibrancy absolutely exists. But it remains unattainable to so many people because they're not making the right decisions and life choices.

If your brain is foggy and you're exhausted, why? How did you get here in the first place? What choices and decisions have you made that led you to today?

We know these are tough questions to ask yourself. We know holding up that mirror and owning our decisions is some bitter medicine. The last thing we want to do is shame or discourage you or make you feel guilty about your past. Quite the opposite.

We want you to feel *empowered* to overcome your exhaustion by making *different* decisions. Because that is what it will take regardless of the underlying causes. Until you change your behaviors, until you make other choices about how you live your life, the energy and vitality you dream of will never be yours.

We can give you all the remedies and solutions in the world, all the tips and tools and techniques to help restore your energy. But we can't get you there.

You have to get yourself there, and that's all *brain*.

You need inner strength and inner fortitude, a will and determination, because, at first, your brain is not going to be your ally. It has a natural aversion to pain. It will do everything it can to protect what is comfortable and known. To the brain, that's safe.

The unknown, the uncomfortable, the new and different behaviors—even if they're healthier—seem dangerous. We're willing to bet there are already topics you've read that have triggered your brain to say, "Not today, Devil." Maybe it was the need to exercise for 15 minutes a day. Maybe it was shutting off devices an hour or two before bed. Maybe it was eliminating sugar and processed foods and carbs. Maybe it was switching personal care products or adding a water filter.

Whatever "it" was, understand that resistance is your brain pushing against making changes. You will not *feel* like doing the remedies we're recommending. You will *feel* too tired. You will *feel* too down. It can take a lot to convince your brain to say no to those three glasses of wine at night, and instead say yes to sitting on the floor and meditating.

Yet different decisions and a new lifestyle are what it will take to get you out of exhaustion.

If your brain will fight you, what can you do? You start small. It's behavior modification that we're talking. You pluck the low-hanging fruit, and you start making the changes that you know you can make and stick with for at least two weeks, preferably a month.

From there, you add another behavior, another new choice. Slow and steady is how you retrain your brain to trust the healthier choices. Before you know it, you will be on the other side of this exhaustion mess in ways you can't imagine.

There's no way around this. To get your brain working right, all your systems have to start firing right. Then, and only then, will your brain have the energy it needs to light up and help you make better decisions. From there, it's an upward spiral.

Energy Remedy Bonus: Call In Herbal Reinforcements

While there is no such thing as cure-all supplements, there are some that can help support a healthy brain. Some of the most popular include:

Turmeric. Turmeric reduces inflammation, detoxes the liver and brain, balances out the microbes in your intestines, and improves memory and cognitive function. Yeah, it's that kickass. You can add turmeric to curries, soups, and even smoothies.

Eleuthero. Eleuthero is great for mental clarity, focus, reducing fatigue, and boosting your energy. It's also known to stabilize blood sugars. You do have to make sure you're taking the right amount. It's a stimulant, so if you take too much, it can make you a little jittery.

You can take small amounts every day for no more than six weeks. Then give yourself a break on it for two to three weeks.

Gingko Biloba. At Dr. Datis Kharrazian's practice, the most effective botanical to use for brain inflammation is gingko biloba, which improves blood flow and blood circulation in the brain.[8] This isn't a new remedy. The leaves of the beautiful gingko tree have been used for centuries to increase blood circulation to the brain. Recent scientific trials are even showing it can be used to help people with cognitive decline and improve their brain function.[9] That's a win in our book.

Gotu Kola. Used for thousands of years in India, China, and Indonesia, gotu kola is known for rejuvenating energy and balancing the nervous system, helping to reduce anxiety and stress. It also helps with mental alertness.

Bacopa. Another important herb in Ayurvedic medicine, bacopa is used to sharpen the mind and help with memory. It's also used to treat anxiety, and it may reduce inflammation. It's often available in pill or powder that you can mix into hot water to make tea.

SOLUTION

Frank's brain wasn't getting the energy it needed to function properly, so he had to make some pretty big lifestyle and dietary shifts to bring back the light. First, he changed his diet, opting to eat more organic vegetables and fruits and more healthy fats like avocados, olive oil, and fish.

He also brought back exercise into his daily life. He used to love jogging, but as his hours creeped up, he had let his exercise slip. Regardless of his busy schedule, he carved out an hour a day for cardio, which helped him manage his anxiety and stress. Finally, Frank stopped work at 6 P.M. At first, he didn't know how he'd get through his workload, but in two weeks, he noticed he could concentrate longer and his work quality improved. His brain felt like it was firing again too. He was seeing the trends and making connections on the funds to invest in.

To his surprise, his brain became more efficient and more powerful when he gave it a break. Things turned around so dramatically for him that within the year, he got a promotion, which eventually led to him running his own hedge fund. Today, Frank continues his hard stop on work each night and remains committed to giving his brain the rest it needs.

PERSONAL CHALLENGE

For one week, give yourself a sanity break during work hours. Once every hour, give yourself permission and make time to walk away from your work, move your body, and/or slow down your mind. For three minutes, do body weight squats, stretch, close your eyes and meditate, do deep breathing exercises, dance, laugh . . . what you do doesn't matter. All that matters is you take a break, give your mind a rest, and bring some peace and lightness into your life.

CHAPTER 9

Spiritual Health

Shawn lived a clean, healthy life. He and his wife had been married for 12 years, and they had three kids. He and his wife didn't talk, go out, or have sex as much as they used to, but hey, they were both busy with careers and raising a family, and that's how marriage with kids was supposed to be.

Shawn ate a pretty balanced diet and stayed active by biking, weight training, and hiking. His financial house was in good shape too, and he didn't feel the stress that a lot of his buddies who were overextended did.

The only black mark he could find was his job, but he felt guilty complaining about it. Shawn was an accountant for an insurance company. His father had been an accountant, so he grew up believing he should be one too. Shawn was also really good with numbers, so the job was easy for him.

There wasn't anything "wrong" with his job. It was just dreadfully boring. But he told himself to suck it up, that he was lucky to have a job that paid him well and offered full benefits. In this economy, what more could he ask for?

Overall, life was pretty good for Shawn, which was why he couldn't figure out why the hell he was so exhausted. Every day felt like a slog, and he felt empty and dull inside. On the weekends, he would take a two-hour nap. Sometimes, just making the kids pancakes was tiring.

At night, after his wife went to sleep, Shawn had taken to playing video games late into the night and whenever he had some downtime. It was his way to unwind and relax, but it had started to interfere with his sleep, keeping him up as late as 1 A.M.

Shawn was feeling so blah that he eventually went to talk with his doctor, who told him it was normal to slow down once a guy his age had kids and a career. His doctor ran some tests, but they all came back in normal ranges. Shawn didn't have any underlying diseases, and he didn't seem depressed. Although there were no obvious signs for his exhaustion, still he felt this lifelessness and he didn't like it.

THE PROBLEM

Go with a physical or mental illness to any native healing tradition around the world, and they don't just hand you some herbs. First, they'll insist on going deeper, meaning spiritually, to find what's off with your *spirit* or *soul*.

If you're in South America, healers often use plant medicine to shake up your internal world. They'll use plants like ayahuasca or huachuma to alter your state of consciousness. Their goal is to challenge your ego and to challenge the beliefs that have created your external world, so that all that's left of you is the real essence of who you are.

If you're in North America and working with indigenous people, they'll often use sweat lodges. It's not plants but heat that cranks up the intensity around you, often bringing out disturbing thoughts that have been lurking in your psyche. These can be negative beliefs about yourself, sabotaging fears about how weak you are, and possibly even past traumas.

Whether you're in South America, North America, or another part of the world, the goal is the same: to pull out your spiritual essence and shake the lower soul to the surface so it can be witnessed and released. Once out of the way, you become a blank slate that's receptive to healing.

The real question is: *What is healing?*

If you're trying to patch up a construct of who you think you are (the storefront defense mechanisms that bolster your fragile narrative), then it likely won't work. You have to heal at your core.

This may sound super intense and way outside your comfort zone, but it works. We've seen many people helped through these ancient ceremonies, which have been used for centuries, possibly longer. We've even sat through these ceremonies ourselves. They've kicked our asses, but in a good way.

While we can't give you any psychedelic plants, and we certainly don't have a sweat lodge to stick you in, we're still going to try to shake up your inner world with the one tool we can wield: *our words*.

In this chapter, we hold nothing back, while challenging everything. This chapter is meant to stir you, shake up your ego, and inspire you to question your religion and beliefs, the meaning and purpose of your life, why you need energy, who you're giving that energy to in your relationships, and who you *think* you are versus the *truth* of who you are.

We want to be direct and candid, because this chapter is the secret. It's the plot twist. It's what this game of life is all about.

Since the beginning, we've walked you through how to ignite your energy from the outside in by using your diet and nutrition, your gut and immune system, sleep and exercise, your adrenals and brain, and so much more. You do these things, and you'll feel better. You'll get a jolt.

But the fastest and best way for you to get over your exhaustion is to ignite your energy from the *inside out*.

All the stuff you've done so far was about building up enough energy so you can stay warm through the dark cold night, until you realized the energy you have been seeking has always been inside of you. That energy is your spirit. It's your soul patiently waiting for you to wake up, to spark the flame, to feed the fire, and then to tap into its infinite energy.

Deep down inside, you know that the broken world that you've lived in and the game you've tried to play are broken. You know this world isn't right. You know this isn't how life is supposed to be. You are not supposed to feel drained and exhausted all the time.

You don't have to fit into that world anymore. You can let yourself wake up by igniting your inner flame.

But we can't light it for you. We can only spark it, and that's our hope. We know what it's like to feel dead inside. The miracle is that no matter how far gone you might think you are, you can rekindle your inner flame and feed the fire at any moment, at any time, no matter your age, no matter what challenges you've faced or are facing.

The power to ignite and stoke your inner fire lies solely with you.

As you make this journey, be open-minded and open-hearted. Be brave. Be courageous. Be true to yourself and your spirit.

When you are true to who you really are, then the broken world that has dragged and drugged you through life will fade away. You will be left walking through this life filled with abundant energy.

THE ENERGY DRAINS

Energy Drain #1: You Don't Know Your Purpose

It's pointless to have high-octane fuel in your tank if you have no idea where you're going or who's at the wheel. Why do you need energy?

It's like gassing up a car with no destination in mind. How many times can you drive around the block? What's the point of the ride?

There once was a nurse who claimed she only slept an hour or two each night. Most people thought that she was lying, and so researchers at a university set out to study her. They thought they'd catch her catnapping.

She turned the tables on them. After two weeks of following her around, the researchers were exhausted. They returned and said she was for real and it was almost impossible to keep up with her. She was the most positive person they'd ever met. She was all about service and living a very caring, compassionate lifestyle. Turns out, all she wanted to do was help others.

She defied science and reason that said people needed at least eight hours of restorative sleep. She needed two hours, at most. What was recharging her? Where was she getting her energy? It was her faith and deep connection to her purpose. She believed there was a reason for her being born and put on this planet, and it was to care for and help other people. It was this *je ne sais quoi* that researchers couldn't explain or understand.

It sounds like she had become what South American indigenous tribes call a *hollow bone*. A hollow bone means there is no ego at play, so the person has become a pure channel for the Universe. When this happens, that person shines *with* the light of the Universe from the inside out, and they become unstoppable. It's what the saints were thought to have become.

There is nothing that will put you on fire, in a good way, like finding the reason you were put here on this earth. When you find this, you find a fountain of endless, unlimited energy that you draw from. People who have something, some purpose, some meaning to live for, tend to live longer, be healthier, and have more energy and vitality.[1]

We know we're talking some pretty lofty aspirations here, and it's by no means easy to become this clear channel for the Universe. But what an intention to set, and we both know from experience, when you find that purpose, you light up.

We're both pretty aligned with knowing why we're here. We know we're meant to help people heal. We know our gifts and talents. We're creative, we're strong communicators, and we have a genuine zest for showing people how to course correct their lives. Knowing and tapping into this meaning and purpose gives us so much juice.

There are days and weeks where we work like thieves. It's not a problem. We will work into the wee hours of the night because we're so mission-aligned that our bodies can find that extra gear. Sometimes it feels like there's a larger force at play.

When you're aligned with your highest ideals, you will find energy reserves you had no idea you possessed. But when you're not dialed in to your purpose, when your mind and body aren't in agreement with your life and how you're spending your energy, you'll have a hard time getting up to face your day.

Energy Drain #2:
You Have Nothing Bigger to Believe In

Meaning and purpose often go hand in hand with religion, spirituality, and belief systems. If you don't believe your life has meaning, if you don't believe there is a purpose to your being here in this time and space, if you don't believe there's a bigger picture, then what's the point?

Without any sense of meaning, life can easily become dull and pointless.

No offense to the atheists out there, but given who the two of us are this shouldn't come as a surprise—*subscribing to the belief that we're just skin-and-bones meat robots is a pretty scary, limiting, and energy-sucking way to live.* The research is in, and the verdict is undeniable—religion and spirituality can have therapeutic effects, whether we're talking about reducing depression, anxiety, exhaustion, or some combination.

If you believe in a higher power, if you believe there is something more to this life, and some purpose to it, then you have a greater chance to live longer (which goes hand in hand with increasing your energy levels). It doesn't matter whether that belief is connected to an organized religion like Islam, Judaism, Catholicism, or to a faith like Hinduism, or a belief and philosophy like Buddhism or Daoism.

It's not the label that matters. It's just having the belief in something bigger that can give you an energy boost.

Is any of this higher power stuff true? We don't know. No one does for sure. Personally, we believe there is something bigger going on in this world that moves the universe and animates all living creatures, plants, animals, insects, and trees alike. We've both had experiences that have shown us the magical interconnection of all life—the deep connection of all life itself. It's a powerful place to be, and once you've witnessed it, it's hard to deny what you've experienced.

But even if that isn't the case, even if the lights go out forever when the final curtain falls, we'd rather trick our brains into believing in something bigger. If that will help us live longer, be happier, be better husbands, fathers, friends, sons—people—then we'll gladly take that placebo pill every day.

Energy Drain #3:
You're Giving Your Energy to Toxic Relationships

The relationships in your life can be a source of energy and really recharge you, or they can drain you. You could do everything else right, but if you're trapped in a toxic relationship, your energy will be completely zapped and drained. There's no compensating for shitty friends, no matter how many chia-seed, magnesium infusions you shoot into your veins.

There are two ways to drink energy in the universe. One way is vertically. It's the path of the mystic or saint, the yogi or the shaman. This is a person whose inner light is so pure, so strong, and so connected to the pulse of the universe that it fuels their very being. They take energy in through heaven and earth and are filled with vibrancy.

The second way is horizontally from plants and animals. This is literally eating food, but it also includes taking or giving energy on a psycho-emotional level with the people in our lives. We are exchanging our energy with people every day, but there are some people who will suck the life force from us.

These are *toxic relationships*. You could have one with your spouse, partner, parent, boss, family member, co-worker, or friend.

Whether we like it or not, each one of our relationships adheres to a spoken or unspoken agreement or contract. These rules of engagement dictate how we behave toward one another, and if they're not crafted in accordance with the good old highest ideals we mentioned earlier, you're going to have challenges.

It's time to take stock of the three to five most important people in your life and start asking some hard questions (don't worry, we've listed out the questions for you in the Remedies section) about whether this relationship, as it currently stands, is fueling or poisoning you.

Energy Drain #4:
You Don't Know Who (or What) You *Really* Are

In Chinese medicine "The Three Treasures" is a belief about the three energies inside each of us that build and sustain life.

Jing is your primordial essence. It's like the mojo you were born with. You can help to bolster it throughout life by doing practices like qigong and through living a clean, healthy lifestyle. You can't get more of it. You work with what you have.

Qi is the energy of life. It translates as "life force," and it flows through your body. Everything in the world has qi. It also gets activated by your jing. It's the energy we're talking about in this book. Qi flows between our organs, fuels our muscles, and powers our life. Everything in life needs energy as a currency.

In Chinese medicine, it's believed that your qi can get depleted. Resting, eating certain foods, exercising, sleeping, and reducing stress are ways to restore it. It's also believed that your qi can get stuck. That's what acupuncture focuses on—opening the channels in the body so your qi can flow easily and unobstructed.

Shen is the spirit, or what in the Western Hemisphere we may call the soul. It's what guides our deeper meaning and place here on the planet, ushering our bodies and energy forward toward a higher purpose. The process of using jing to power qi is all about illuminating shen, so we can wake to who we truly are—a flame that burns the Eternal fire of all that is.

The metaphor for The Three Treasures is a candle. Jing is the wax, qi is the fire, and shen is the glow around the flame.

When you balance the three energies by living a good, clean life, the outcome is self-realization. Self-realization is knowing and connecting with who you really are. When you do this, you live a fulfilled, meaningful life complete with everything we talked about—meaning and purpose, belief in a higher power, and loving and connected relationships.

Most of us are like candles that burn too fast. We eat the wrong foods, we don't get enough sleep or exercise, we're not detoxing or managing stress, and so our flame burns too hot and too quick, and the wax melts everywhere. If you burn down the candle too fast, you don't get the self-realization or the chance to live a fulfilled life. That's an unhealthy "burn rate."

Now, instead imagine this beautifully still candle and flame that gives off a gentle yet penetrating glow, an aura. The point of life is to create this glow around ourselves that helps us illuminate and see the light through the darkness. The point is to activate our consciousness, to wake up, and become a light unto ourselves.

The real question is, how do you burn in the universe? Do you glow?

We're going to get real spiritual with you for a second, so strap in. In the ancient religions like the Kabbalah, and the original Merkabah, which was Egyptian, and the hundreds of others, the sun was the source of all life. In these ancient traditions, an enlightened human was reborn a star.

What is a star? It is your consciousness understanding the essence of *who you are* to such an extent that you combust at the end of this life and become a star yourself.

You become a brilliant indestructible light unto the universe, and that's really *the* point. It's not about running around, making kids, and buying Porsches. This game of life is about becoming the brightest, most activated version of yourself. It's about becoming a still candle, and eventually building up enough power to ignite as a sun (which is a star), so you can be a beacon of light in your world and community.

It's about connecting deep within to the true essence of who you are, to *what* you are. Anything that leads you away from your self-realization, that has you forgetting who you really are, will leave you exhausted.

Personal Quest (Pedram)

I am the son of immigrants. My parents were born in Iran. My father went to school in Germany before he and my mother brought my sister and me to America. As a kid, I'd finish my homework and goof off in my bedroom. My father, like many immigrants who have sacrificed for their kids, would open my door and want to know, "What's going on here?"

I'd tell him I was done with my homework. He'd stare at me for a second and then tell me to go study something else. I'd be like, "What do you mean go study something else? I'm eight!"

At a very young age, I learned the trick was to always look busy. I'd finish my homework and then start doodling at my desk, so when Dad came in and asked what I was doing, I could happily say, "Math!" and he'd be so proud and be like, "That's great!"

My dad was a fantastic dad. But this experience laid the foundation for a very flawed operating system in me that I have to work to unwind. It's hard for me to relax, especially in front of my wife. I'll catch myself sitting on the couch for five minutes, but as soon as she walks into the room, I'm up and have to show her I'm doing something productive. Can't have her thinking she married some deadbeat!

This is ridiculous. I'm 44 years old. I'm a doctor and Daoist priest. I studied with the Dalai Lama. I run two companies. I'm a documentary filmmaker. I'm a *New York Times* best-selling author, and I can't show my wife that I'm relaxing because I'm afraid she'll think I'm slacking off? When I lay it out like that, it sounds stupid, yet this is what's going on in my head.

It would absolutely drain my energy and leave me exhausted if I didn't notice these thoughts, and if I couldn't separate them from who I really am.

This is why I meditate and practice martial arts. I'm constantly zoning in on stilling my mind so that I can separate my bullshit from that deeper part of myself that's filled with energy and peace. I've practiced this stuff for decades, and I *still* have to constantly turn the mirror on myself, asking, "Who's saying that?" I have to actively practice relaxing with my wife and being open with her about my wounds.

Is it worth it? Absolutely. It's these daily practices that keep my energy flowing, so I have the juice I need to live my life.

TESTS

Your spiritual health is very personal and unique. Only you can assess its health and whether this part of your life needs some nurturing and adjusting. Unlike the other tests we've described, there is no blood work, saliva, or stool test that can determine whether you're operating at the highest level.

Instead, what we've done is created a series of questions designed to help you self-reflect and assess your spiritual health. Make sure you're in a quiet spot. Don't overthink the answers. Go with your immediate answer, and don't overanalyze the response. This isn't about going deep to ask "Why?" questions.

It's about helping you to see clearly, to feel clearly, to sense clearly what's happening in your inner world. Keep your answers in mind as you read through the Remedies.

1. Do you believe you have a purpose in this life?

2. Do you know what your purpose is in life?

3. Do you feel connected to this purpose?

4. Do you believe in something bigger than yourself?

5. Do you want to believe in something bigger?

6. Consider the primary relationships in your life. Do you feel these people love, support, and encourage you?

7. Do you feel belittled, demeaned, or judged in any of these relationships?

8. Do you feel safe in these relationships, where you can say or do anything and you would still be loved and supported?

9. Are there thoughts left unsaid or feelings left unexpressed to the people you're closest with that need to be released?

10. Do you feel you have a relationship with yourself?

11. Do you trust your instincts and intuition?

12. Do you act kind to yourself, practicing self-care?

13. Do you, or can you, forgive yourself for mistakes?

14. Do you hold yourself to unrealistic expectations?

15. Do you feel excited, joyful, and grateful for your life?

16. Do you have a regular practice that strengthens your spiritual health?

17. Do you want to have a more regular or a more robust practice?

THE ENERGY REMEDIES

Energy Remedy #1: Learn Your Purpose

"I find that people who live on purpose, who live in their passion, who follow their bliss, generally are energized and magnetized by the quality of life they're living. They're not just living their life; they're living their soul," shared Sachin Patel, a functional medicine practice success coach. "If we can get people to find their purpose, if we can get people to follow their bliss, if we can get people to be magnetized by their day, then they tap into this kind of unmeasurable energy. It's not something that we can see on lab work. It's this innate force that drives us. It's the force that drives everything in the universe."[2]

What Sachin described sounds incredible, and we don't know anyone who would say no to living their soul. The trick is figuring out what that passion and purpose is. If you're unsure, then ask yourself, *What was I put here on this earth to do? What are my gifts and talents? What do I love doing?* This may or may not be your profession. It could be a hobby. It could be an interest. It could be a volunteer opportunity. It could be raising your kids. It could be how you walk through the world every day interacting with strangers.

Finding your meaning and purpose isn't always connected to the term "success" as we culturally define it in the West. It's not about gaining some level of name recognition or making oodles of money. Maybe you get both. Maybe you don't.

What matters is you discover and stand in your truth, knowing that *this*—whatever this is—is what you were born to do.

That's for you to find, not for us to tell you. But, speaking from experience, we know how charged you will become when you find your meaning and purpose. We hope and pray you do.

Another tool is to make a list of your passions. What are you interested in? What lights you up? What moves you? Is there a social, environmental, or humanitarian cause you feel passionately about? Keep the inquiry simple. Ask yourself, *What action or activity would make me truly happy right now, in this moment?* or *If I could be anyone, doing anything, what would that be?*

Or you could go straight to the *Braveheart* approach (our personal fav) and ask yourself, *What cause, idea, or community would I give my life for?* This may seem dramatic, but the world needs heroes and heroines now more than ever.

If you already know what that passion is, but for whatever reason it got placed in a drawer, consider how you can bring it back into your life in small, sustainable ways. Just taking tiny steps toward returning to your passion and purpose will immediately bring a sense of life and energy to your every breath.

Energy Remedy #2: Discover Your Beliefs

Finding something to believe in will help give your life meaning and purpose amid the daily grind that can be stressful, annoying, and defeating.

Maybe it's becoming part of a cause. We live in a time where social justice, environmental issues, and economic challenges are taking center stage. People are joining and becoming a part of bigger movements. Maybe you're called to become more engaged in your community, helping to rebuild and revitalize where you live.

Maybe discovering your beliefs is about tapping into a religion or faith. Religions and faith can be complicated. We're not going all in on any one religion, faith, or belief system. We're not saying to bow down and become a Christian, a Buddhist, a Hindu, or any other organized religion or faith. Nor do we necessarily think running back to your parent's place of worship is the answer.

If you want to find religion or dial in to a more faith-based way of living, be discerning. Any religion that attempts to shame you, wants to limit you, or tells you that you're going to hell unless you play by their rules should immediately go on your watch list. Religions and faith should uplift you. They should encourage you to shine, not try to dim your light.

Energy Remedy #3: Evaluate Your Relationships

We only have one life to live. Who are you giving your energy to? Who are you surrounding yourself with? Are you surrounded by positive or negative people? Are you surrounded by people who lift you up or drag you down?

When you're evaluating where your exhaustion is coming from, it's worth looking at the people in your life.

About 15 years ago, Nick started studying and working with shamans. Along this journey, it became very easy for him to realize what relationships were worth keeping and which ones he needed to let go of.

Once he began awakening to the realization of this bright light inside of himself, and that it was his birthright to shine, it became almost offensive when someone tried to take it away.

The fact is that some people, intentionally or not, will try to dim your light.

This isn't a rally cry for you to call up a divorce lawyer or to cut off all contact with your parents (although that may have to be the boundary you set). First, it means getting brutally honest with yourself about what relationships in your life lift you up, and which ones drag you down.

Grab a sheet of paper and draw a line down the center. In the left-hand column write, "Dragging Me Down," and in the right-hand column write, "Uplifting Me." Next, start naming names.

With your "Dragging Me Down" list complete, now you're ready to determine which relationships to keep and work on, and which ones to rewrite or let go.

We know we're simplifying this. We could write an entire book on toxic relationships. The goal here is to just figure out if toxic relationships may be the source for your exhaustion woes.

If you decide a semi-toxic relationship is worth keeping, then you've got some work to do. It means you're going to have to set better boundaries. That may mean you need to start saying no or expressing your thoughts, emotions, and needs more. This may require getting counseling or other professional support. Expect it to take time to fully course correct.

Whatever it takes, do it. It's worth the investment.

In the meantime, here are two practices you can use immediately to offer some relief.

1. Review Unspoken Contracts

Fair warning, whatever relationships you want to keep will likely require some serious work. They'll require some tough conversations. You'll have to be open and honest with your feelings.

When you enter a relationship there is always some sort of unspoken contract that develops. Nick and his wife check in on their unspoken contracts regularly. They're like, "Wait a second. I never told you I was willing to compromise in that part of my life. I can't do that. Can we talk about it? What can I do for you instead?"

They're very open communicators and committed to problem solving together. They're also very introspective and cast the light back on themselves. You need to know what you need as individuals and what you need as partners.

2. Cord Cutting

Maybe you realize you have a relationship that needs releasing. A popular way to let it go peacefully is to practice cord cutting. It's a way to release the energetic connection between you and another person. This is something used in many different healing traditions around the world.

You want to sit quietly, close your eyes, and visualize an ex, a friend, a parent, a boss, or someone you feel has been draining your energy. Imagine a cord connecting the two of you, and then cut it. How you cut it is up to you. Imagine using scissors, an ax, or a saw, or dissolving it, burning it, or using whatever tool or form that feels most comfortable.

As you're cutting this cord, imagine telling the person that you release them with love and wish them well, and that you no longer wish to be energetically connected. Repeat this process as often as you need.

Energy Remedy #4: Find the Light Within

Your power, your energy, your vitality comes from the stillness within. It comes from becoming that still candle and flame.

But the chaos within can stop you from becoming this still, powerful candle.

This is where meditation can be your friend. It is the best tool to return to your center, to remember who you really are, and to become a sun unto the universe. The gap between wanting and knowing you need to meditate, and being able to meditate, can be pretty wide.

If you're someone who thinks, *Oh my god, I close my eyes and I can't silence my mind, it's too hard,* well, yeah, it's going to be hard. Too bad. This is where you start. Now, sit down, close your eyes, focus on your breath, *shut up,* then repeat.

Do this until you realize how *ridiculous* your inner voice is, how loud it is, how busy it is, how absolutely tumultuous it is between your two ears. If you can realize that this chaos is what becomes your life, and it becomes who you are as a person, then you will be able to separate who you think you are from who you really are.

We don't expect you to meditate for two hours every day. Like everything else, start small. Start with one step that you can take. If meditation hasn't been your thing, start by just sitting comfortably, legs crossed, on the floor, with your eyes closed for five minutes in the morning. Set a timer and go.

If five minutes is too much, then start with two. Do this for a week every morning, and then add another two- to five-minute session at night. It doesn't matter what emotion, memory, vision, words, or thoughts come up. Don't censor. Don't try to control anything. Just let whatever rises up, rise up.

If you want a more advanced meditation technique, ask, "Who am I?" See and hear the response. When you think you have an answer, ask the question again. Ask, "Who is asking this question?"

There will never be a final answer, just more depth to uncover. The answer has little to do with who you think you are and a lot more to do with finding the *essence* of who you really are. That being, that radiant infinite spirit, who has never lacked energy—that's the being you seek in meditation.

Energy Remedy Bonus: Build Your Integrity

The translation of Genesis is "As I speak, I create." If every morning you get up and say, "Today is finally the day I'm going to the gym," or "Today is finally the day I'm going to eat well," but then you don't, it's like you've betrayed yourself. When you don't follow through on your word to yourself, you have compromised your integrity.

When we don't honor ourselves, we create a rift between ourselves and our souls. It proves to the chaotic voice within that we're losers, that we're incapable of following through, and that what we say doesn't matter.

Your word and the actions that mirror it are all you have. One of the first steps toward rekindling your soul is to stop compromising your word to yourself. Don't say you'll do something that you can't do.

We keep banging the steel drum of taking small steps and making small commitments in large part for this reason. We want you to rack up victories, to see and feel success, and to prove to yourself that you're capable of great things. Every time you set and keep your word, you build your honor and you quiet that chaotic voice inside. This is another great way to silence that talking head that's been living rent-free in your head.

All it takes is one act, one push up, one green smoothie at a time. This is also how you build your fire. When you get a small fire going, you don't just drop a huge log on the flame. That will snuff it out. You lay some kindling and smaller pieces, let them catch, and slowly you build up the fire, the heat, and the intensity. Once it's going, it's raging.

Before you realize it, you will have built up your inner fire, and you will be amazed by how much more energy you have to get things done.

SOLUTION

Shawn had done everything right. His exhaustion wasn't from diet or exercise or sleep or toxins or anything we've previously described. It was from his job and his relationship with his wife.

Shawn knew he didn't like his job. He just had no idea how much of his life force it was stealing from him. Reversing Shawn's exhaustion took some time, but it started with him getting real and raw with himself. He wasn't prepared to make a drastic career change. Instead, he decided to try to use his skills in service of his passions.

Shawn was passionate about environmental causes and the great outdoors, so he began searching for accounting positions at organizations and businesses working in the environmental space.

He also looked for opportunities to get involved with local organizations that were connected to the environment. He and his family loved hiking, so he decided to become a hike leader, organizing outings that his family and others in their community enjoyed on the weekends. He fell in love with planning, organizing, and leading these hikes. And for a bonus energy boost, he met some amazing people who became fast friends.

Just realizing how passionate he was about the environment and outdoors and taking a couple small steps really reinvigorated Shawn and helped him start reversing his exhaustion mess.

He also talked with his wife about reconnecting with her and curbing his video game playing. With the help of a therapist, Shawn realized he craved greater intimacy and connection with his wife. When he asked to talk with her about it, he was surprised to learn she missed that part of their relationship too, and she felt just as exhausted.

They agreed to start scheduling time together. They put time on their calendars for sex and intimacy and talking. Shawn cut back on his video game playing. He still played sometimes on the weekends and once or twice during the week, but he also made time at night for him and his wife to spend together.

Within a couple of months, Shawn's energy and vitality for life returned. But it wouldn't have if he hadn't stopped to take stock of what was happening on the spiritual front of his life and being.

PERSONAL CHALLENGE

Grab a timer, find a quiet, distraction-free, comfortable spot on the floor or a chair where you can put both feet on the ground, and meditate.

For one week, we challenge you to meditate for five minutes in the morning, as soon as you get up, and five minutes at night, preferably before you go to bed.

Your mind may resist at first. Your thoughts may be loud. You may have visions and images flashing. Whatever comes up—a thought, an emotion, an image—just notice it. You don't have to do anything.

You do this for a week, and you will find that the noise starts to get quieter. You may even start looking forward to your meditating time, possibly even extending it from 5 minutes to 10. Before you know it, it can easily become a 30-minute practice every day that you start looking forward to. You may add a meditation session at lunch or wake up early just to give yourself some extra time.

CHAPTER 10

Thriving in a Broken World

Shortly after Pedram moved to Utah with his family, his wife asked him about their power bill. It had doubled. He figured it was some heating coils or something connected to living in a colder climate than L.A. and called the handyman and asked him if they should change out some heating coils. The handyman said no way; those wouldn't cause that much of an energy drain. But he did notice that the downstairs fridge was running really hot because the fan wasn't working right.

He was spot on. That one faulty appliance had caused the electric bills to soar and sucked money out of Pedram's pocket.

The moral here: Where are you losing energy? Go back and ask yourself what part of your life is stealing your energy.

This may be the end of our exhausted road trip, but it's not the end of your journey. It's just the beginning. Hopefully, you've already tried some remedies and are feeling a little bump in your energy. We've given you the very best advice on exhaustion from some of the world's top experts. But it wasn't individualized.

Now it's up to you to take this information and use it to transform your life, and frankly, your world. It's time to find where you're leaking energy, fix the drains, and get your energy economics right.

As you go forward, try to keep some of the big themes of *Exhausted* in mind:

Self-care isn't selfish; it's the right thing for you and your loved ones

What holds many people back isn't lack of information. It's the gap between knowing what they should do, and actually doing it. We really do understand. You're pushed and pulled in so many different directions. You have so many people relying on you, asking for your time, attention, and energy.

You want to be there for them.

You want to be the best mother or father you can, the best spouse or partner, the best boss or employee, the best friend or sibling. There's nothing wrong with wanting this or for caring about the well-being of the people in your life. But what happens far too often is you put yourself last.

Taking care of yourself is not a selfish act. It's an act of love and caring. When you recharge and refuel your energy, it means you can show up more present and more engaged with the people you love, the work you're doing, and the life you're living.

Make one small tweak, and build on that

Don't try to be a hero or heroine by doing everything, or taking on more than you can handle. Like we've said, no one does everything. Start small and build up. Tweak one area of your life, then another, then another. Before you know it, you will have built a solid foundation for your energy.

You have the power to heal

It's very easy to get caught up in listening to the "right" advice. You're bombarded with experts. It's hard to know what and whom to listen to. This isn't about discarding or distrusting experts. We all need them. But there's also a place for knowing and listening to your body. If something doesn't feel right, trust your instincts. That goes for this book and the collected advice we've shared.

If you need it, get medical help
We believe you have the ability to heal your exhaustion. And we're also keenly aware that some people need more support than a book can provide. You may need to seek help from someone in the medical community, and that's probably going to be someone other than your general practitioner.

This isn't to take away from the excellent care that Western medical doctors provide. They certainly play an important role in health, wellness, and healing. But they've also been trained to identify a disease, drop a label on you, and treat you with drugs. Exhaustion is a huge catch-all label with many different roots.

You need someone who can look more holistically at your body to evaluate how it's functioning. Talk to a functional medical professional. If you're nervous about the cost, talk to them. It's not easy being open about finances, but many professionals care about ensuring evaluations and treatments are effective and workable on every level—including financial. It can feel like you need to take out a loan just to run some of the tests. Don't do that. Talk with your doctor first. (And if you feel pressured into something, get the hell out of that office and find a new medical ally.)

Whomever you seek, find someone who will take the time to work with you who will help you test and monitor your levels, and who can help you determine the right supplements and dosages to take.

Doctors and other health practitioners can be some of your greatest allies on this quest. Use them. You don't have to go it alone.

This is a journey, so keep going
Fixing your exhaustion does not happen overnight. It does not happen in one week, and it may not even happen in one month. For both of us, it took about six months to get our energy flowing again. For some people, it can take less time, sometimes more. Be patient. Be steadfast. Focus on one change, one day at a time.

And don't you dare give up. Don't you dare stop fighting to reclaim your energy. It is your birthright. You are meant to be a star that shines brightly. Become that star, and don't stop until you do. Even if it takes your entire life—and it probably will—keep going.

There is light at the end of the tunnel

Right now, it may seem so far away, maybe even impossible, to regain your energy and vitality. You didn't lose your energy overnight, and you're probably not going to regain it overnight either. But little by little, day by day, tweak by tweak, you'll start to get to the other side. People heal from exhaustion. They regain their zest and zeal for life. They learn how to manage their energy levels, so they have the energy they need for their commitments. You, too, can do this. We know you can.

WHICH DREAM DO YOU CHOOSE?

When you get your energy levels back, does it mean that life starts throwing you rainbows, unlimited sunshine, unicorns, and ticker-tape parades? Does it mean you just get to kick back on the beach sipping mai tais? *Hell no.*

Life will always challenge you. You'll still have kids to parent; a job to do; a career to build; a spouse to connect with; friends, siblings, and parents to spend time with; communities to engage with; and whatever else you fill your days with.

The difference is you now have the energy to do it all, and to live your life. When you have the energy to meet your commitments, then you're able to handle whatever curveballs life throws at you with more grace, patience, fortitude, and peace.

The first step in any new direction is always the hardest. You just took that by reading this book. Now take the next one. Before you know it, you will be on the other side of this exhaustion mess and experiencing life in ways you couldn't imagine. Your body is strong. It's resilient. The more you take care of it, by feeding it healthy and clean foods, by letting it rest and sleep at night, by exercising it and building its lean muscles, the more it will take care of you.

The stronger your body is, the better prepared it will be to defend against any invaders and threats. You'll also find that when your energy is humming, you can drop in a late night every now and again, you can have an extra glass of wine occasionally or a cheeseburger and fries, and those little indulgences won't tank you. Oh, you'll probably feel them, but you'll bounce back. And the unexpected stresses that will certainly pop up, well, guess what? You'll manage them with greater ease too.

We're rooting for you. We believe in you. We know that you have the power to restore your energy. You and only you, can reverse your exhaustion. You can do this.

In fact, you have to. Look around. The world has gone mad. It's exploding. Everyone is fighting. The climate is collapsing. The world—our planet—is falling apart. Mother Earth—this third rock from the sun we call home—is exhausted too.

The questions before you are simple: Do you want to live in a world of exhaustion, where you keep running while overworked and stressed out? Do you want to exist in a universe where your energy and life force is always depleted? Or do you want to slow the hell down, restore your energy, use it with purpose, and live in balance?

Chaos and exhaustion or peace and vitality?

You choose your dream, so which one do you want to keep projecting?

We know our answer.

What will you choose?

Endnotes

Chapter 1

1. Dr. David Perlmutter, interview with the authors, August 2019.

Chapter 2

1. "How Many Calories Are in One Gram of Fat, Carbohydrate, or Protein?" USDA National Agricultural Library, accessed December 30, 2019, https://www.nal .usda.gov/fnic/how-many-calories-are-one-gram-fat-carbohydrate-or-protein.

2. "Treating Sugar Addiction Like Abuse: QUT Leads World-First Study," QUT, April 7, 2016, https://www.qut.edu.au/news?news-id=103307.

3. Ari Whitten, interview with the authors, August 2019.

4. Shan, et al., "Trends in Dietary Carbohydrate, Protein, and Fat Intake and Diet Quality Among US Adults, 1999–2016," *Journal of the American Medical Association* 322, no. 12 (September 24, 2019): 1178–1187. doi:10.1001/ jama.2019.13771.

5. Ibid.

6. Ibid.

7. "Iron," National Institutes of Health, Office of Dietary Supplements, accessed November 16, 2019, https://ods.od.nih.gov/factsheets/ Iron-HealthProfessional/.

8. Steiber, A., Kerner, J., and Hoppel, C. L., "Carnitine: A Nutritional, Biosynthetic, and Functional Perspective," *Molecular Aspects of Medicine* 25, no. 5–6 (October–December 2004): 455-73. https://www.ncbi.nlm.nih.gov/ pubmed/15363636.

9. Westman, et al., "Implementing a Low-Carbohydrate, Ketogenic Diet to Manage Type 2 Diabetes Mellitus," *Expert Review of Endocrinology & Metabolism*, 13, no. 5 (September 2018): 263-272. https://www .ncbi.nlm.nih.gov/pubmed/30289048.

10. Maggie O'Neill, "The Keto Diet Might Prevent Migraines—Here's What You Need to Know," *Health*, April 29, 2019, https://www.health .com/condition/headaches-and-migraines/keto-diet-migraine.

11. Eric Kossoff, "Ketogenic Diet," Epilepsy Foundation, October 2017, accessed February 24, 2020, https://www.epilepsy.com/learn/ treating-seizures-and-epilepsy/dietary-therapies/ketogenic-diet.

12. Dr. David Perlmutter, interview.

13. Shubhroz, G., and Satchidananda, P., "A Smartphone App Reveals Erratic Diurnal Eating Patterns in Humans That Can Be Modulated for Health Benefits," *Cell Metabolism* 22, no. 5 (November 2015): 789–798. https://www.ncbi.nlm.nih.gov/pmc/articles/PMC4635036/.

Chapter 3

1. "Fast Facts About the Human Microbiome," The Center for Ecogenetics and Environmental Health, January 2014, https://depts.washington.edu/ceeh/downloads/FF_Microbiome.pdf.

2. Ibid.

3. S. B. Eaton, "The Ancestral Human Diet: What Was It and Should It Be a Paradigm for Contemporary Nutrition?" The Proceedings of the Nutrition Society 65, no. 1 (February 2006):1-6. https://www.ncbi.nlm.nih.gov/pubmed/16441938.

4. Katherine D. McManus, "Should I Be Eating More Fiber?" Harvard Health Publishing, February 27, 2019, https://www.health.harvard.edu/blog/should-i-be-eating-more-fiber-2019022115927.

5. Ibid.

6. Ibid.

7. Dr. Datis Kharrazian, interview with the authors, August 2019.

8. Ari Whitten, interview.

9. Dr. Datis Kharrazian, interview.

10. Untersmayr, E., and Jensen-Jarolim, E., "The Role of Protein Digestibility and Antacids on Food Allergy Outcomes," The Journal of Allergy and Clinical Immunology 121, no. 6 (June 2008): 1301–1310.

11. Jennifer Couzin-Frankel, "Can Antacids Boost Allergy Risk?" Science, July 30, 2019, https://www.sciencemag.org/news/2019/07/can-antacids-boost-allergy-risk.

12. Cassady, et al., "Mastication of Almonds: Effects of Lipid Bioaccessibility, Appetite, and Hormone Response," *The American Journal of Clinical Nutrition* (March 8, 2009). http://ucce.ucdavis.edu/files/datastore/608-11.pdf.

13. Dr. Kellyann Petrucci, interview with the authors, August 2019.

Chapter 4

1. Dr. Heidi Hanna, interview with the authors, August 2019.

2. Rottensteiner, et al., "Physical Activity, Fitness, Glucose Homeostasis, and Brain Morphology in Twins," *Medicine and Science in Sports and Exercise* 47, no. 3 (March 2015): 509–18. https://www.ncbi.nlm.nih .gov/pubmed/25003773.

3. Ari Whitten, interview.

4. Ibid.

5. Ibid.

6. Ben Greenfield, interview with the authors, August 2019.

7. Dr. Stephanie Estima, interview with the authors, August 2019.

Chapter 5

1. Dr. David Perlmutter, interview.

2. Dr. Datis Kharrazian, interview.

3. "1 in 3 Adults Don't Get Enough Sleep," Centers for Disease Control and Prevention, February 16, 2016, https://www.cdc.gov/media/releases/2016/ p0215-enough-sleep.html.

4. Stuart Quan, "What Is the Magic Sleep Number?" Harvard Health Publishing, October 29, 2015, https://www.health.harvard.edu/blog/ what-is-the-magic-sleep-number-201509168280.

5. Rubin Naiman, "Dreamless: the Silent Epidemic of REM Sleep Loss," *ANNALS of The New York Academy of Sciences* (August 15, 2017). https://nyaspubs .onlinelibrary.wiley.com/doi/abs/10.1111/nyas.13447.

6. Cirelli, C., and Tononi, G., "The Sleeping Brain," *Cerebrum* 2017 cer-07-17 (May 1, 2017). https://www.ncbi.nlm.nih.gov/pmc/ articles/PMC5501041/?report=classic.

7. Dr. David Perlmutter, interview.

8. Beccuti, G., and Pannain, S., "Sleep and Obesity," *Current Opinion in Clinical Nutrition and Metabolic Care* 14, no. 4 (2011): 402–12. doi:10.1097/ MCO.0b013e3283479109.

9. Maya Allen, "Is It Bad to Eat Before Bed? Nutritionists Answer," The Thirty, May 4, 2019, https://thethirty.whowhatwear.com/is-it-bad-to-eat-before-bed.

10. Ananya Mandal, M.D., "Caffeine Pharmacology," News Medical Life Sciences, updated Feb 26, 2019, accessed December 6, 2019, https://www.news-medical .net/health/Caffeine-Pharmacology.aspx.

11. Markham Heid, "What's the Best Time to Sleep? You Asked," *TIME*, April 27, 2017, https://time.com/3183183/best-time-to-sleep/.

12. Christensen, et al., "Direct Measurements of Smartphone Screen-Time: Relationships with Demographics and Sleep," *PLoS ONE* 11, no. 11 (2016): e0165331. https://journals.plos.org/plosone/article?id=10.1371/journal .pone.0165331.

13. Christopher Bergland, "Late-Night Smartphone Use Often Fuels Daytime Somnambulism," *Psychology Today*, January 18, 2017, https:// www.psychologytoday.com/us/blog/the-athletes-way/201701/ late-night-smartphone-use-often-fuels-daytime-somnambulism.

14. Cassie Bjork, interview with the authors, August 2019.

15. Dr. Stephanie Estima, interview.

16. Ananya Mandal, M.D., "Caffeine Pharmacology," News Medical Life Sciences, updated Feb 26, 2019, accessed December 6, 2019, https://www.news-medical .net/health/Caffeine-Pharmacology.aspx.

Chapter 6

1. David Ewing Duncan, "Chemicals Within Us," *National Geographic*, accessed January 3, 2020, https://www.nationalgeographic.com/science/ health-and-human-body/human-body/chemicals-within-us/.

2. Ibid.

3. Dr. Robert Rountree, interview with the authors, August 2019.

4. James Hamblin, "The toxins that threaten our brain," *The Atlantic*, March 18, 2014, https://www.theatlantic.com/health/archive/2014/03/ the-toxins-that-threaten-our-brains/284466/.

5. Andrew Weil, "Are Flame Retardants Toxic?" Dr.Weil.com, October 9, 2014, https://www.drweil.com/health-wellness/balanced-living/healthy-home/ are-flame-retardants-toxic/.

6. Axel, et al., "Human Health Implications of Organic Food and Organic Agriculture: A Comprehensive Review," *Environ Health* 16, no. 111 (2017). https://www.ncbi.nlm.nih.gov/pmc/articles/PMC5658984/#CR79.

7. Średnicka-Tober, et al.,"Higher PUFA and n-3 PUFA, Conjugated Linoleic Acid, A-Tocopherol and Iron, but Lower Iodine and Selenium Concentrations in Organic Milk: A Systematic Literature Review and Meta- and Redundancy Analyses," *The British Journal of Nutrition*, 115, no 6. (Mar 28, 2016): 1043-60. https://www.ncbi.nlm.nih.gov/pubmed/26878105.

8. Dani Williamson, interview with the authors, August 2019.

9. Yvette Brazier, "How Does Bisphenol A Affect Health?" *Medical News Today*, accessed November 20, 2019, https://www.medicalnewstoday.com/ articles/221205.php.

10. Mark Wilson, "The Air You Breathe at Home Might Be Worse than the World's Most Polluted Cities," *Fast Company*, April 11, 2019, https://www.fastcompany .com/90332899/the-air-you-breathe-at-home-might-be-worse-than-the-worlds -most-polluted-cities.

11. "About Dental Amalgam Fillings," U.S. Food and Drug Administration, accessed January 6, 2020, https://www.fda.gov/medical-devices/dental -amalgam/about-dental-amalgam-fillings.

12. Dr. Afrouz Demeri, interview with the authors, August 2019.

13. Houlihan, et al., "Body Burden: The Pollution in Newborns," Environmental Working Group, July 14, 2005, https://assets.ctfassets.net/t0qcl9kymnlu/ 2GVUmYpZCgu6iuSiKEUY4m/9ccbb2938066649259c634806957d499/Body _Burden_in_Newborns.pdf.

14. Ibid.

15. "Identifying and Reducing Environmental Health Risks of Chemicals in Our Society: Workshop Summary," *National Academies Press*, October 2, 2014, https://www.ncbi.nlm.nih.gov/books/NBK268889/.

16. Ibid.

17. Ibid.

18. "Drink Tap Water," City of New York, accessed November 16, 2019, https:// www1.nyc.gov/site/greenyc/take-action/drink-tap-water.page.

19. "State With the Most Fluoridated Water," Fluoride Alert, March 2, 2016, http:// fluoridealert.org/news/states-with-the-most-fluoridated-water/.

20. "Is Flouridated Drinking Water Safe?" *Harvard Public Health*, Spring 2016, https://www.hsph.harvard.edu/magazine/magazine_article/ fluoridated-drinking-water/.

21. Ibid.

22. Austin Price, "Organic Diet Significantly Reduces Risk of Pesticide Exposure," UC Berkeley Public Health, February 19, 2019, https://publichealth.berkeley .edu/news-media/school-news/organic-diet-significantly-reduces-risk-of -pesticide-exposure-new-study-shows/.

23. Dr. David Perlmutter, interview.

24. Sheryl Huggins Salomon, "What Is Glutathione? A Detailed Guide to the Antioxidant and Supplement," *Everyday Health*, January 4, 2019, accessed November 30, 2019, https://www.everydayhealth.com/diet-nutrition/diet/ glutathione-definition-uses-benefits-more/#foodsources.

25. "Urbanization and Water Quality," USGS, accessed November 30, 2019, https://www.usgs.gov/special-topic/water-science-school/science/urbanization -and-water-quality?qt-science_center_objects=0#qt-science_center_objects.

Chapter 7

1. Dr. Meghan Walker, interview with the authors, August 2019.

2. Dr. Heidi Hanna, interview.

3. "Adrenal Insufficiency Diagnosis," University of California San Francisco, accessed January 6, 2020, https://www.ucsfhealth.org/conditions/adrenal -insufficiency/diagnosis.

4. Dr. Heidi Hanna, interview.

5. Dr. Anna Cabeca, interview with the authors, August 2019.

6. Dr. Darin Ingels, interview with the authors, August 2019.

Chapter 8

1. Ferris Jabr, "Does Thinking Really Hard Burn More Calories?" *Scientific American*, July 18, 2012, https://www.scientificamerican.com/article/thinking-hard-calories/.

2. Dr. Datis Kharrazian, interview.

3. Dr. David Perlmutter, interview.

4. Jaime Ducharme, "Americans Are Some of the Most Stressed-Out People in the World, a New Global Survey Says," *TIME*, April 25, 2019, https://time.com/5577626/americans-stressed-out-gallup-poll/.

5. Dr. Datis Kharrazian, interview.

6. Dr. Leigh Erin Connealy, interview with the authors, August 2019.

7. Qing Li, "Effects of Forest Bathing on Cardiovascular and Metabolic Parameters in Middle-Aged Males," *Evidence-Based Complementary and Alternative Medicine* 2016 (July 14, 2016). https://www.ncbi.nlm.nih.gov/pubmed/27493670.

8. Dr. Datis Kharrazian, interview.

9. Napryeyenko, O., and Borzenko, I., "Ginkgo Biloba Special Extract in Dementia with Neuropsychiatric Features: A Randomised, Placebo-Controlled, Double-Blind Clinical Trial," *Arzneimittelforschung* 57, no. 1 (2007): 4–11. https://www.ncbi.nlm.nih.gov/pubmed/17341003.

Chapter 9

1. Dennis Thompson, "Have a Purpose, Have a Healthier Life," *U.S. News*, December 10, 2019, https://www.usnews.com/news/health-news/articles/2019-12-10/have-a-purpose-have-a-healthier-life.

2. Sachin Patel, interview with the authors, August 2019.

Index

A

F

Acknowledgments

This book is a brain trust. It's filled with ideas, insights, and stories from some of the greatest minds and healers we've had the privilege to work with and learn from. We owe much debt and gratitude to the people who made this book what is it. Maryna Allan, Bree Argetsinger, Debra Atkinson, Robyn Benson, Summer Bock, Maggie Berghoff, Michael Breus, Cassie Bjork, Trevor Cates, Anna Cabeca, Jill Carnahan, Jodi Cohen, Joe Cohen, Leigh Erin Connealy, Amanda McQuade Crawford, Amy Day, Afrouz Demeri, Maru Davila, Gwen Dittmar, Erin Elizabeth, Udo Erasmus, Stephanie Estima, Keesha Ewers, Jake Fratkin, Ben Greenfield, Darin Ingles, Heidi Hanna, Mark Hyman, Tero Isokauppila, Datis Kharrazian, Rushelle Khanna, Kasie Kines, Susan Lovelle, Deborah Matthew, Joe Mercola, Tom O'Bryan, Reshma Patel, Sachin Patel, David Perlmutter, Kellyann Petrucci, Warren Phillips, Valencia Porter, Shelese Pratt, Sarah Rattray, Tom Rofrano, Robert Rountree, Christine Schaffner, Isabel Sharker, Mariza Snyder, Meghan Walker, Debora Wayne, Ari Whitten, Dani Williamson, Doni Wilson, Magdalena Wszelaki, Eric Zielinski, and Sabrina Ann Zielinski—*thank you* for being a part of this project and for sharing your wisdom with us.

To our film crew who helped us research, organize, shoot, and produce the hundreds of hours of interview footage. Lorenzo Phan, Mileen Patel, Courtney Donnelly, Sean Rivas, Carl Lindahl, and Dave Girtsman—there is no way we could have done this project without you. Thank you all!

To Amanda Ibey, thank you for bringing our vision for *Exhausted* to life. Because of you, it turned out even better than we could have imagined or hoped. To Courtney Donnelly and Tom Malterre, thank you for reviewing manuscript drafts and offering invaluable suggestions.

Finally, we are blessed to work with the incredible team at Hay House. Reid Tracy, Patty Gift, Lisa Cheng, and everyone on the Hay House team, thank you all for believing in this project from the beginning and supporting us every step of the way.

About the Authors

Dr. Pedram Shojai is a man with many titles. He is the founder of Well.org and the *New York Times* best-selling author of *The Urban Monk, Rise and Shine, The Art of Stopping Time*, and *Inner Alchemy*. He is the producer and director of the movies *Vitality, Origins*, and *Prosperity*, and he has also produced several documentary series, including *Interconnected, Gateway to Health*, and *Exhausted*. In his spare time, he's a Taoist abbot, a doctor of Oriental medicine, a kung fu world traveler, a fierce global green warrior, an avid backpacker, a devout alchemist, a qigong master, and an old-school Jedi bio-hacker working to preserve our natural world and wake us up to our full potential. You can visit him online at www.theurbanmonk.com.

Nick Polizzi is a producer and director of feature-length documentaries about holistic alternatives to conventional medicine. He is the founder of The Sacred Science, director of the feature documentary by the same name, and author of the book based on the film. Nick's mission as host and executive producer of the docuseries *Remedy: Ancient Medicines for Modern Illness* is to honor, preserve, and share these powerful, evidence-based healing technologies with those who have been failed by modern medicine and the system as a whole. Ever since he cured himself of a debilitating illness at age 25 using a traditional therapy, he has been traveling the world and documenting forgotten healing methods. You can visit him online at thesacredscience.com.

Hay House Titles of Related Interest

YOU CAN HEAL YOUR LIFE, the movie,
starring Louise Hay & Friends
(available as a 1-DVD program, an expanded 2-DVD set,
and an online streaming video)
Learn more at www.hayhouse.com/louise-movie

THE SHIFT, the movie,
starring Dr. Wayne W. Dyer
(available as a 1-DVD program, an expanded 2-DVD set,
and an online streaming video)
Learn more at www.hayhouse.com/the-shift-movie

▪

*EMF*D: 5G, Wi-Fi & Cell Phones: Hidden Harms and
How to Protect Yourself,* by Dr. Joseph Mercola

*OWN YOUR SELF: The Surprising Path beyond Depression, Anxiety, and
Fatigue to Reclaiming Your Authenticity, Vitality, and Freedom,*
by Kelly Brogan

*THE POWER OF VITAL FORCE: Fuel Your Energy,
Purpose, and Performance with Ancient Secrets of Breath
and Meditation,* by Rajshree Patel

*REGENERATE: Unlocking Your Body's Radical Resilience through the
New Biology,* by Sayer Ji

All of the above are available at your local bookstore,
or may be ordered by contacting Hay House (see next page).

▪

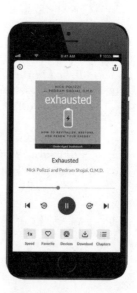